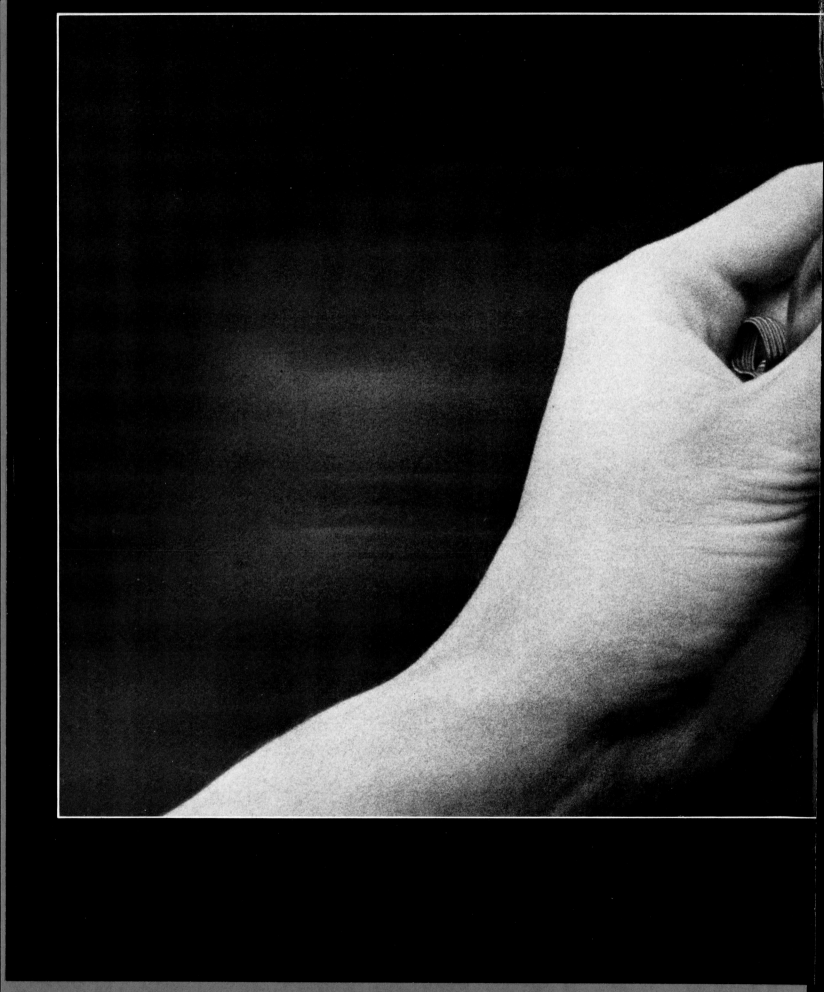

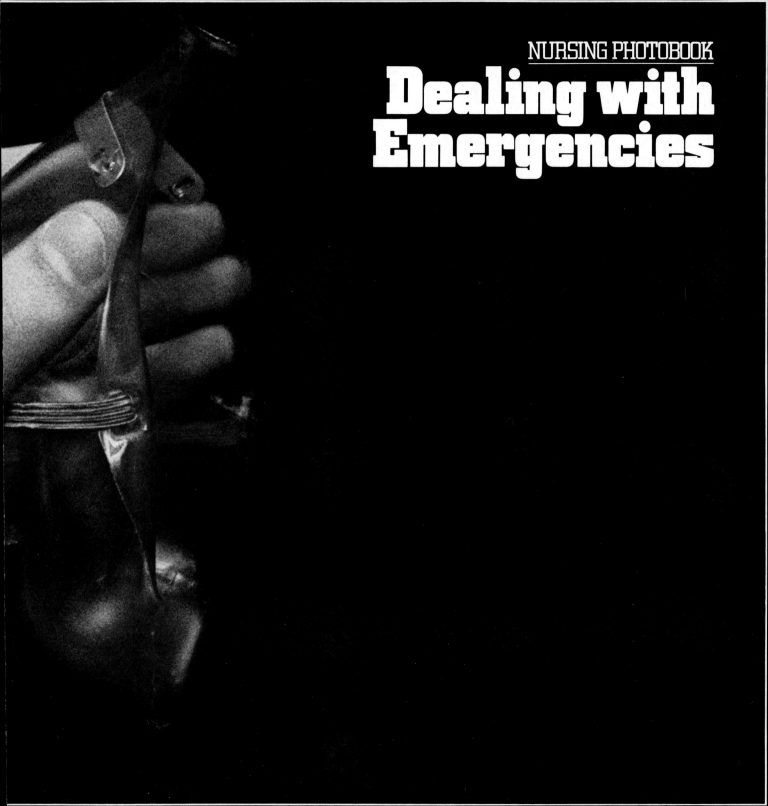

NURSING PHOTOBOOK

Dealing with Emergencies

NURSING83 BOOKS™

NURSING PHOTOBOOK™ **SERIES**
Providing Respiratory Care
Managing I.V. Therapy
Dealing with Emergencies
Giving Medications
Assessing Your Patients
Using Monitors
Providing Early Mobility
Giving Cardiac Care
Performing GI Procedures
Implementing Urologic Procedures
Controlling Infection
Ensuring Intensive Care
Coping with Neurologic Disorders
Caring for Surgical Patients
Working with Orthopedic Patients
Nursing Pediatric Patients
Helping Geriatric Patients
Attending Ob/Gyn Patients
Aiding Ambulatory Patients
Carrying Out Special Procedures

NURSING SKILLBOOK® **SERIES**
Dealing with Death and Dying
Reading EKGs Correctly
Managing Diabetics Properly
Assessing Vital Functions Accurately
Helping Cancer Patients Effectively
Giving Cardiovascular Drugs Safely
Giving Emergency Care Competently
Monitoring Fluid and Electrolytes Precisely
Documenting Patient Care Responsibly
Combatting Cardiovascular Diseases Skillfully
Coping with Neurologic Problems Proficiently
Nursing Critically Ill Patients Confidently
Using Crisis Intervention Wisely

NURSE'S REFERENCE LIBRARY® **SERIES**
Diseases
Diagnostics
Drugs
Assessment
Procedures

Nursing83 **DRUG HANDBOOK**™

NURSING PHOTOBOOK™ **Series**

PUBLISHER
Eugene W. Jackson

EDITORIAL DIRECTOR
Jean Robinson

CLINICAL DIRECTOR
Barbara McVan, RN

**Intermed Communications
Book Division**

DIRECTOR
Timothy B. King

DIRECTOR, RESEARCH
Elizabeth O'Brien

DIRECTOR, PRODUCTION AND PURCHASING
Bacil Guiley

Staff for this volume

BOOK EDITOR
Patricia Reilly Urosevich

CLINICAL EDITOR
Mary Horstman Obenrader, RN

ASSOCIATE EDITORS
Sanford Robinson
Patricia Russo
Richard Samuel West

PHOTOGRAPHER
Paul A. Cohen

ASSOCIATE DESIGNERS
Lisa Gilde
Linda Jovinelly Franklin

DESIGN ASSISTANT
Lorraine Lostracco Carbo

ASSISTANT PHOTOGRAPHER
Thomas Staudenmayer

EDITORIAL/GRAPHIC COORDINATOR
Doreen K. Stowers

COPY EDITOR
Barbara Hodgson

EDITORIAL STAFF ASSISTANT
Evelyn M. James

ART PRODUCTION MANAGER
Wilbur D. Davidson

ARTISTS
Darcy Feralio   Robert H. Renn
Diane Fox   Sandra Simms
Terry Jackson   Louise Stamper
Deborah Lugar   Ron Yablon
Robert Perry

TYPOGRAPHY MANAGER
David C. Kosten

TYPOGRAPHY ASSISTANTS
Ethel Halle
Diane Paluba

PRODUCTION MANAGER
Robert L. Dean, Jr.

PRODUCTION ASSISTANT
M. Eileen Hunsicker

ILLUSTRATORS
Dimitrios N. Bastas   Robert Jackson
Jack Crane   Cynthia Mason
Jean Gardner   John R. Murphy
Tom Herbert   Bud Yingling

SERIES GRAPHIC DESIGNER
John C. Isely

COVER PHOTO
Seymour Mednick

**Clinical consultants
for this volume**
Jeanne Dupont, RN
Head Nurse
Massachusetts Eye and Ear Infirmary
Boston

Julieta D. Grosh, MD, FACS
Surgical Director, Emergency Department
Temple University Hospital
Philadelphia

Barbara Krajewski, RN
Intensive Care Unit
Crozer-Chester Medical Unit
Chester, Pennsylvania

Amended reprint, 1983
© 1980 by Intermed Communications, Inc., 1111
Bethlehem Pike, Springhouse, Pa. 19477
All rights reserved. Reproduction in whole or part by
any means whatsoever without written permission
of the publisher is prohibited by law.
Printed in the United States of America.

PB-060483

Library of Congress Cataloging in Publication Data

Main entry under title:
Dealing with emergencies.

(Nursing Photobook)
Bibliography: p.
Includes index.
1. Emergency nursing   I. Intermed
Communications, Inc.   [DNLM: 1. Emergencies—
Nursing text.   WY154 D279]
RT120.E4D42   610.73'61   80-11450
ISBN 0-916730-20-4

Contents

Contributors

At the time of original publication, these contributors held the following positions.

Judith Ann Bailey is the nurse coordinator of the Regional Trauma Center, University Hospital, University of California Medical Center, San Diego. She received her BSN from San Diego State University and her MBA from National University, also in San Diego. Ms. Bailey is a member of the American Association of Critical Care Nurses, and the American Trauma Society.

Phyllis A. Hagerty received her RN from Beebe Hospital School of Nursing, Lewes, Delaware. She is a staff nurse at the Crozer-Chester Burn Treatment Center, Chester, Pennsylvania. Ms. Hagerty is a member of the American Burn Association, and the American Nurses' Association.

Catherine Lodge Hawkes is currently on leave from her position as clinical instructor of maternity nursing at Chestnut Hill Hospital, Philadelphia, Pennsylvania. A graduate of the Hospital of the University of Pennsylvania, she earned her BSN from the University of Pennsylvania, Philadelphia. She is an MSN candidate at the University of Pennsylvania. Ms. Hawkes is a member of the American Nurses' Association, Childbirth Education Specialists, and the Nurses' Association of the American College of Obstetricians and Gynecologists.

Carol Horton is a graduate of the Pennsylvania Hospital School of Nursing, Philadelphia, and is currently enrolled in the external degree program at St. Joseph's College, North Windham, Maine. Ms. Horton is the critical care coordinator at Wake County Medical Center, Raleigh, North Carolina.

Elaine S. Jackson received her RN from the St. Francis Hospital School of Nursing, Wilmington, Delaware. She is a staff nurse at the Crozer-Chester Burn Treatment Center, Chester, Pennsylvania. Ms. Jackson is a member of the American Burn Association, and the American Nurses' Association.

Betty L. Landon, one of the advisers on this book, is the assistant director of nursing for critical care units and the emergency department at Temple University Hospital, Philadelphia, Pennsylvania. She graduated from the Bellevue School of Nursing, New York City, and received her BA from the University of Redlands (California). Ms. Landon is studying for her MA at Temple University.

Cheryl Larkin is a graduate of the Montgomery Hospital School of Nursing, Norristown, Pennsylvania. She is the head nurse of the emergency department, Montgomery Hospital, Norristown.

Shirley Heaton Marshburn, also an adviser on this book, is the nursing supervisor of the emergency department at Winter Park (Florida) Memorial Hospital. A graduate of St. Margaret's Hospital School of Nursing, Montgomery, Alabama, she is a BSN candidate at Southern Missionary College, Orlando, Florida. Ms. Marshburn is a member of the Emergency Department Nurses' Association.

Patricia O'Brien received her BSN from Villanova (Pennsylvania) University and her MSN from the University of Pennsylvania, Philadelphia. At the time of this writing, Ms. O'Brien was a musculoskeletal clinical specialist at Thomas Jefferson University Hospital in Philadelphia. She is a member of the American Nurses' Association, and Sigma Theta Tau.

Suzanne Tracey Zamerowski is a clinical instructor of obstetric nursing at Villanova (Pennsylvania) University. A graduate of St. Francis Medical Center School of Nursing, Trenton, New Jersey, she received her BSEd from Temple University, Philadelphia (Pennsylvania). Ms. Zamerowski earned her MSN from the University of Pennsylvania, Philadelphia. She is a member of the Nurses' Association of the American College of Obstetricians and Gynecologists, the American Nurses' Association, and Sigma Theta Tau.

Introduction

Challenge. Isn't that what emergency nursing is all about? Are you ready to meet that challenge whenever or wherever it occurs? When seconds count, your advance preparation pays off, because you'll have to instinctively recall all your knowledge, skills, and experience *stat*.

Obviously, that's a big order for you to fill. But no one said emergency nursing was easy. We, in the PHOTOBOOK Department, understand your predicament so well that we designed this book especially for you. It'll provide you with those vital skills you need when a moment's hesitation on your part may jeopardize your patient's life.

For example, do you know how to use a defibrillator correctly? How to manage a sucking chest wound? How to help the doctor insert an anterior/posterior nasal pack? If you don't, you'll discover how in this PHOTOBOOK. It contains step-by-step instructions for these important procedures, complete with clear, quality photographs.

But these aren't the only nursing procedures we've highlighted in this PHOTOBOOK. Consider these: How to insert a Foley catheter…How to apply rotating tourniquets…How to perform a gastric lavage. We've also included some at-the-scene emergencies in which your expertise may be needed. On those carefully prepared pages, you'll learn how to help the victim of a diving accident, how to cope with a traumatic amputation, and how to deliver a baby.

What makes this PHOTOBOOK better than other nursing textbooks? We go beyond *words*. We *show* you what you need to know in hundreds of carefully selected photographs. In addition to these photostories, our staff has prepared some illustrated charts covering many common emergencies. Use these highly comprehensive charts to help set your nursing priorities. They've been designed especially to serve in situations when you need a quick, handy reference.

And that's not all this PHOTOBOOK includes. Watch for the eye-catching minidesigns used throughout the book. These logos highlight specific tips and features; for example, patient preparation, troubleshooting equipment, and complications. You'll also find some imaginative patient teaching aids that you can copy for your patients. All these extras make nursing easier, because they sharpen your skill, increase your efficiency, and bolster your self-confidence.

Working nurses from the United States and from Canada have contributed to this special PHOTOBOOK. Sharing their knowledge with you has been their way to help you meet the challenge of emergency nursing. Welcome the opportunity to learn from them. You'll face that challenge wherever you work.

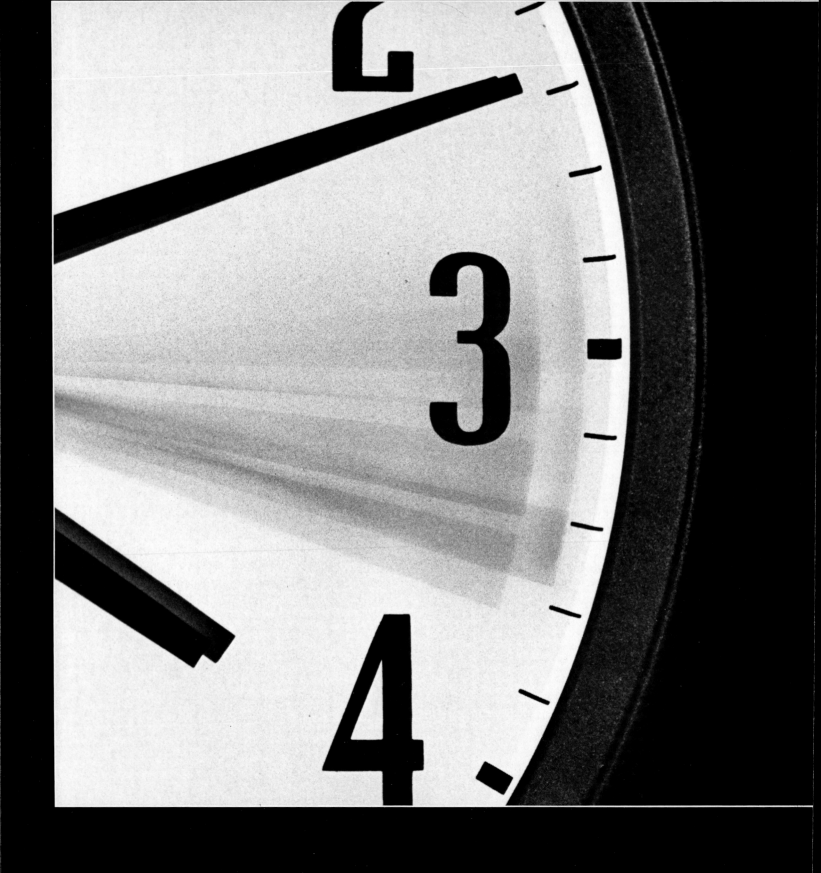

Performing an Emergency Assessment

Assessment

Assessment

In case of an emergency, are you prepared to give prompt and efficient care to a patient whose life is in danger? Do you know how to quickly assess the patient's airway, breathing, and circulation? Can you perform a head-to-toe emergency assessment while taking the patient's medical history?

Throughout this PHOTO-BOOK, we'll show you how to improve your emergency nursing skills. We'll teach you what to do—as well as what *not* to do—when responding to an emergency, whether your patient's on the street, at home, in a doctor's office, or in the hospital.

ABCs of emergency assessment

Suppose you're the first health-care professional at the scene of an emergency. As your first nursing responsibility, perform a 90-second assessment of the patient's airway, breathing, and circulation (ABCs).

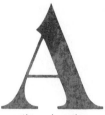

AIRWAY ▷ Check your patient's airway. Look for signs of respiratory distress: gasping, wheezing, cyanosis, and restlessness. If the patient is choking or making crowing noises (stridor), suspect airway obstruction from a foreign body or an acute allergic reaction.
▷ If a foreign body's blocking your patient's airway, try to relieve the obstruction. Open his mouth, using the crossed-finger technique shown below. Then, sweep two fingers of that hand or your other hand deep into his mouth to remove any foreign matter. (For detailed instructions, see page 20.) If this method fails, try giving back blows and abdominal thrusts, as explained on pages 18 and 19.
▷ If you suspect that an acute allergic reaction's responsible for blocking the patient's airway, *call the doctor immediately.*
▷ Is the patient unconscious and supine? If he is, his tongue may have fallen back, occluding his airway. Use the head-tilt maneuver described on page 21 to correct this. *Caution:* Never hyperextend the patient's neck if you suspect a spinal injury; instead, use the modified jaw thrust, described on page 23.

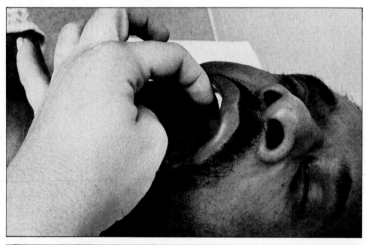

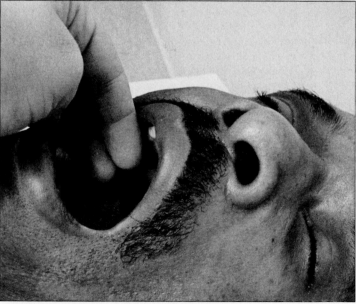

BREATHING ▷ Check your patient's breathing to determine if his respirations are adequate. To do this, put your ear close to his mouth and nose. Can you detect air movement? Now, look at his chest and abdomen. Do you observe a rhythmic rise and fall? What about the quality of his respirations? Is he having trouble breathing? Is he using the accessory muscles in his neck? Remember, dyspnea may suggest myocardial infarction. *Notify the doctor immediately.*

▷ If your patient hasn't started breathing spontaneously after you've performed the head-tilt or the jaw-thrust maneuver, ventilate his lungs immediately, using the mouth-to-mouth technique explained on pages 21 through 23.

▷ If your patient has a mouth injury, or you can't get a good seal because he has no teeth, use the mouth-to-nose technique explained on page 24.

▷ Does your patient have a stoma from a tracheotomy or laryngectomy? Restore his breathing by giving mouth-to-stoma ventilations, as described on page 25.

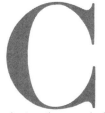

CIRCULATION ▷ Check your patient's circulation by feeling for a pulse in his carotid artery. Does he have neck injuries? Feel instead for a femoral pulse. If no pulse exists, assume his circulation has stopped. Begin cardiopulmonary resuscitation (CPR) immediately. To find out how to give CPR to an adult or child, carefully study the detailed instructions and photos on pages 27 through 30.

▷ Is the patient bleeding? Profuse bleeding, especially arterial, calls for immediate treatment. In most cases, you can control bleeding by applying direct pressure on the wound with a sterile dressing. Or you can apply pressure on the closest pressure point between the wound and the patient's heart. For further details on these and other methods used to control bleeding, see the instructions on pages 36 through 38 and 43.

▷ Internal bleeding may also be present. Suspect it when your patient shows signs of hypovolemic shock (see pages 40 and 41). Keep him warm as you continue to monitor him closely. Then, transport him to a hospital immediately.

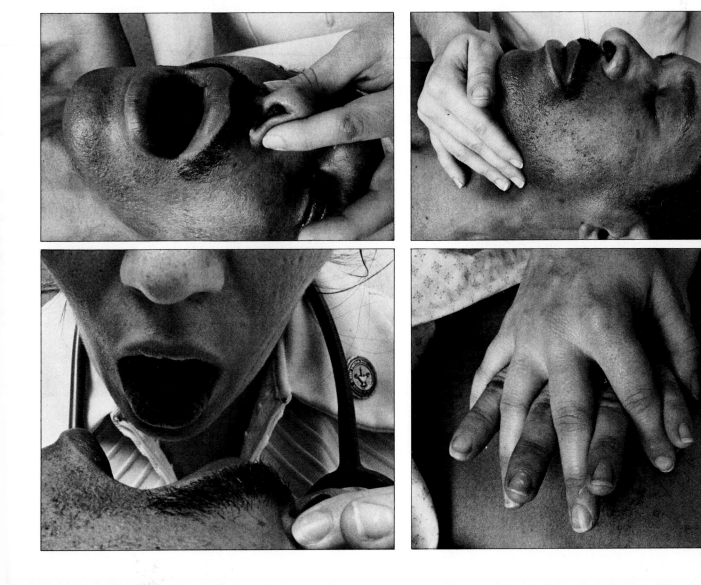

Assessment

How to perform an emergency assessment

After you've checked your patient's ABCs and have attended to any immediate problems, what next? Perform the head-to-toe emergency assessment shown here as quickly and efficiently as possible. Its systematic approach will help you to collect the most information about your patient in the least amount of time. Afterwards, reassess and care for any problems or injuries you've detected.

Important: The digital readouts you'll see at the beginning of each caption are merely guides, not the actual time that's to be spent on each body part.

To begin, assess your patient's general appearance and level of consciousness. Ask yourself these questions: Is he alert and oriented to time, place, and person? Is he restless or combative? Is his speech incoherent or slurred? Does he seem to have trouble understanding or interpreting questions? Are his answers appropriate? Is he unconscious? If so, does he respond to verbal stimuli? Painful stimuli? Is he comatose?

If your patient's not alert and fully oriented, or if he has a head injury or multiple trauma, you'll need to monitor his neurologic signs. In a comatose patient, *unilateral* neurologic deficits (hemiparesis or single dilated pupil) may indicate an intracranial lesion. *Bilateral* neurologic deficits may indicate intoxication or a severe metabolic disorder. (For further details on neurologic deficits, see pages 130 to 132.)

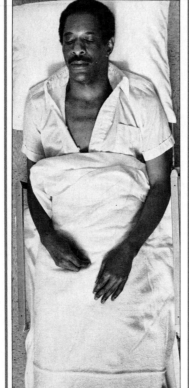

Next, inspect your patient's pupils. Are they equal in size and shape? How do they react to light? (For detailed instructions on performing pupillary checks, see pages 130 to 132.)

As you examine the patient's eyes, look for evidence of trauma (lacerations, contusions), excessive tearing or dryness, or pale or reddened conjunctivae. Tearing and reddened conjunctivae may indicate irritation from a foreign body or infection. Dryness and pallor suggest hypovolemia or a sympathetic nerve lesion. (For additional information, see page 40.)

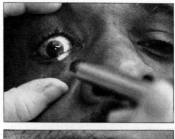

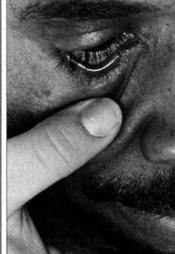

Now, examine your patient's ears, nose, and mouth for possible drainage. If drainage is present, note the color, amount, and consistency. As you examine the patient's face, ask yourself: Is his facial expression symmetrical? Any ptosis? Does his mouth droop on one side? Any circumoral cyanosis? Pallor? Flushing? Are his lips bright red? If they are, suspect carbon monoxide poisoning.

Nursing tip: If your patient's dark-skinned, don't attempt to evaluate skin color changes without first examining his conjunctivae, palms, and soles.

Before you go on, note any facial lacerations, but don't stop to deal with superficial bleeding or you'll risk missing a more serious injury elsewhere.

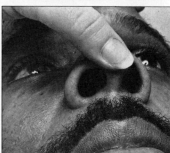

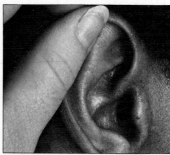

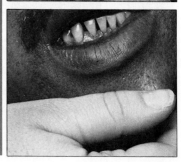

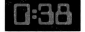

Next, examine the patient's head and scalp, as the nurse is doing in this photo. Carefully look for lacerations, avulsed tissue, deformities, or soft spots that could indicate a depressed skull fracture.

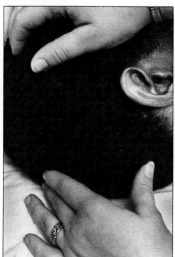

Open your patient's mouth and look inside. To help you see better, use a penlight. Examine his buccal mucosa and under his tongue. See any cyanosis? Inflammation? Bleeding? Check also for loose or missing teeth. Smell your patient's breath, and describe the odor as well as you can in your notes. Suppose the odor is fruity and sweet. This may indicate the presence of acetone, which is a sign of diabetic acidosis.

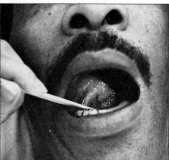

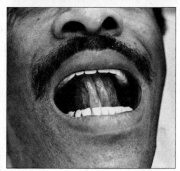

Examine your patient's neck, as the nurse is doing here. Palpate his jugular veins. If they're distended, pulsating, or collapsed, he may have pulmonary or right heart complications. Next, slide your fingers over his suprasternal notch to palpate his trachea. If the trachea's shifted from midposition, check his lung sounds. He may have atelectasis, tension pneumothorax, or a large pleural effusion.

Can you feel crepitus on palpation? If so, suspect subcutaneous emphysema from a fractured trachea, or pneumothorax.

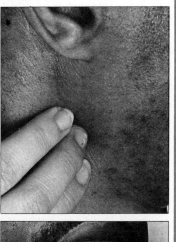

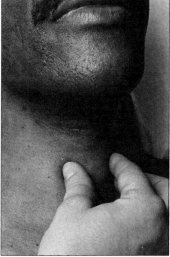

To examine your patient's chest, first remove his clothing, so you won't overlook anything significant. Then, look for lacerations, puncture wounds, deformities, rashes, or scars. If he has a chest wound, note the color, amount, odor, and consistency of any drainage. Ask yourself these questions: Are the patient's chest movements symmetrical? Is he using his accessory muscles to help him breathe? Does his sternum retract during inspiration? Does he need to keep his head elevated to breathe comfortably?

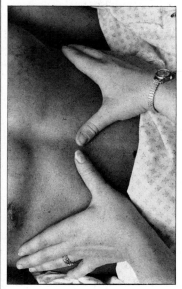

Assessment

Use a stethoscope to listen to your patient's breath sounds, and count his apical heart rate. (To find out exactly how to do this, study the NURSING PHOTOBOOK *Providing Respiratory Care*.) Also, observe the rate and rhythm of his respirations, and document any abnormal patterns; for example, Biot's, Cheyne-Stokes, or Kussmaul's. *Nursing tip:* Is your patient complaining of pain in his left shoulder? If he's had a fall, he may be having *referred* pain from a ruptured spleen.

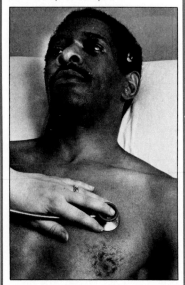

Now, remove any clothing from your patient's abdomen so it won't hinder your assessment. Then, look for distention, obvious masses, lacerations, puncture wounds, or scars. At the same time, assess his skin condition. Look for abnormal pigmentation, lesions, striae, or dehydration signs, like dryness and poor skin turgor. If he has a wound, note the color, amount, odor, and consistency of any drainage. Then, using the stethoscope, listen for bowel sounds. *Important:* Always listen for bowel sounds *before* you palpate your patient's abdomen. Why? Because palpation may stimulate bowel activity and mask the patient's true condition.

Does your patient have abdominal pain? Gently palpate his entire abdomen. Try to distinguish between local and referred pain, spasm, rigidity, and rebound tenderness. If possible, ask him about the nature of the pain: Is it sharp? Shooting? Dull? Constant? Persistent? Intermittent? Does it radiate? How long has it been present? Has he had it before?

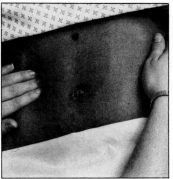

Moving downward, examine the patient's genitals and perineum. Look for lacerations, avulsed tissue, swelling, ecchymosis, or skin lesions. Is there a noticeable discharge? If so, note the amount, color, and consistency. Also, check for urinary or fecal incontinence.

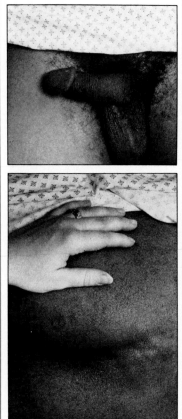

Next, examine your patient's extremities. Among other things, you'll be checking for the five *P*s: pulse, pallor, pain, paresthesia, and paralysis. Start by noting any obvious deformities, such as open wounds, missing digits, or fractures. (For guidelines on assessing fractures, see pages 90 and 91.)

If your patient's conscious, ask: Is he in pain? Can he move his arms and legs? Any impairment of sensation?

Now, check your patient's nailbeds, as the nurse is doing in this photo. Do you see any cyanosis or pallor? Remember, if your patient's dark-skinned, check his palms and soles too. (For more details on how to do this accurately, see the NURSING PHOTOBOOK *Assessing Your Patients*.

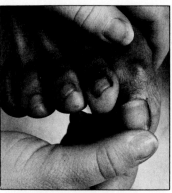

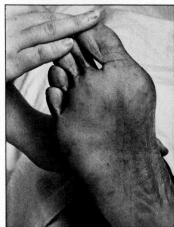

Check your patient's radial, pedal, popliteal, and femoral pulses bilaterally. Compare for rate and rhythm.

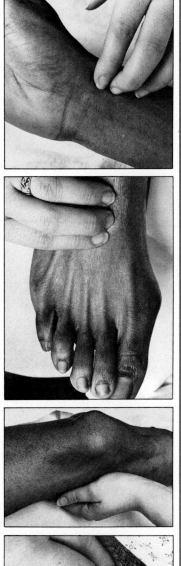

Now, check the patient's blood pressure. Unless something more urgent needs attention, measure his blood pressure in both arms. If he can move, check his blood pressure in his left arm while he's sitting, standing, and lying down.

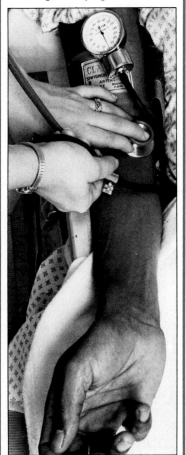

To check for edema, look at your patient's ankles. Do they appear swollen? If so, perform the following test: Gently depress the skin directly over his lower tibia, as the nurse is doing here. If he has pitting edema, the depression made by your fingers will remain. *Remember:* In a bedridden patient, check for sacral rather than pedal edema.

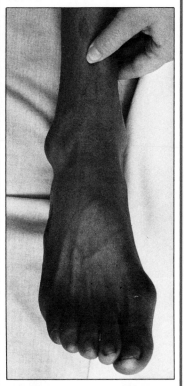

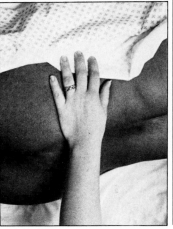

If your patient's condition permits, finish your assessment by turning him, so that you can examine the back of his body from head to toe. Look for lacerations, puncture wounds, hematomas, scars, deformities, unusual pigmentation, or skin lesions. *Important:* Never attempt to turn a patient if you suspect he has a cervical injury or a fractured pelvis; to do so could cause serious, perhaps irreversible, complications.

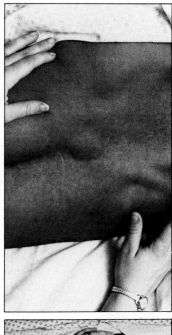

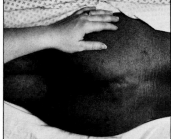

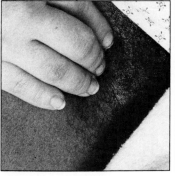

Assessment

Getting the patient's history

While you perform a head-to-toe emergency assessment, take a brief medical history of your patient. To do this properly, tailor your questions to the patient's physical condition.

For example, suppose he's dyspneic? Don't ask questions that require more than a yes or no answer. However, if he's not dyspneic and seems alert and oriented, you can ask open-ended questions like "Have you ever had a pain like this before?" or "How does this pain differ?"

If the patient doesn't seem to comprehend what you're asking, consider the possibility that he's deaf or speaks a foreign language. Locate someone who can act as an interpreter. Or, attempt to communicate with him yourself, using simple gestures.

Never neglect getting an adequate history because you can't communicate with your patient for some reason; for example, if he's unconscious or has a fractured jaw. Instead, gather the information you need from all available resources: ambulance personnel, police officers, witnesses, family members, or previous medical records.

Check to see if your patient's wearing a Medic Alert bracelet or necklace (see page 15 for details). If necessary, search his wallet for a medical identification card. Remember, besides finding out why your patient came to the hospital or clinic, you'll need answers for the following questions: Does the patient have any allergies, diseases, or disorders? How has he been treated for these conditions? Does he take any medications? Who is his regular doctor?

Carefully record your findings on the patient's chart, keeping in mind that your nurses' notes may serve as a data base during his hospitalization. To ensure accurate charting, some hospitals use a data collection sheet like the one shown at the right. A properly filled out data collection sheet provides all health team members with the information they need to care for the patient. Take time to be thorough; don't leave any blank spaces.

Patient Data Base

Name *Griff, Edmund* Age *52* Sex *male*

Date *7/15/79* Time *2 am* Height (Approx.) *5'11"* Weight (Approx.) *216 lbs.*

Allergies *all drugs ending in "mycin"*

Vital Signs:

Blood Pressure *150/102* Temperature *97* Radial Pulse *74*

Apical Heart Rate *98* Respirations *24*

Nursing Observations *flushed, diaphoretic, anxious*

Patient's Chief Complaint *"My chest hurts." "I can't breathe"*

How long have symptoms been present? *1½ hrs.*

Was the patient treated for these symptoms before? Yes *X* No

If yes, when? *6 months ago* Where? *here*

Result *angina pectoris*

Any history of disorder or disease? (include mental) *maternal grandmother had diabetes and heart disease*

Recent Activity *walking up 2 flights of stairs*

Taking any medications? Yes *X* No If yes, what? *nitrol ointment ½" am & pm; Inderal 80 mg QID; Isordil 10 mg ac & HS; Digoxin 0.25 mg O.D.; NTG gr 1/150 SL prn*

State of Consciousness:

Alert? *X* Oriented: Time *yes* Place *yes* Person *yes*

Neurologic:

Pupil check (describe): *pupils equal and reacting to light*

Responsive to painful stimuli? *yes* Unresponsive?

Nursing comments *answers all questions appropriately*

General Appearance:

Pale? *no* Cyanotic? *yes* Nailbeds? *yes* Circumoral cyanosis? *yes*

Flushed? *yes* Jaundiced? *no* Clammy skin? *yes* Cool skin? *yes*

Other? *anxious expression*

Physical deformity? *none*

Prosthesis? *glasses*

Scars? *gallbladder surgery – 1960*

Nursing comments *good hygiene*

Patient's Behavior:

Restless? *yes* Anxious? *yes* Irritable? *no* Hostile? *no*

Depressed? *no* Lethargic? *no* Other?

Nursing comments *somewhat anxious but cooperative*

Patient's doctor *Dr. David Smith*

Who gave this information? *patient and his wife*

Attending nurse *Mary Obenrader, RN*

MINI-ASSESSMENT

Is your patient wearing a Medic Alert™ bracelet or necklace?

What if your patient can't speak or otherwise communicate with you? And what if he arrives in the emergency department without family or friends? How can you get his medical history? See if he's wearing a Medic Alert bracelet or necklace. This jewelry, shown below, displays the following information: the patient's hidden medical condition, his identification number, and a 24-hour emergency phone number.

If it's your responsibility to care for the patient, obtain his complete medical data by calling the emergency phone number. When the operator answers, give her the patient's identification number. The operator will then supply you with the patient's medical history from a computerized file. *Remember:* When you document the patient's medical history on his data collection sheet, be sure you indicate the source.

For free information, write to the Medic Alert™ Foundation, P.O. Box 1009, Turlock, California 95380.

Nurses' guide to assessment pitfalls

After you've assessed the patient and documented your findings, what should you do? Most importantly, avoid drawing hasty—and possibly inaccurate—conclusions about the patient's condition. Never assume you can immediately identify all your patient's problems. And always keep your eyes and ears open for sudden changes in his condition. Study the chart below to avoid some common assessment pitfalls.

If your patient has these signs and symptoms	Don't automatically assume he has this problem	It may also be
Restlessness, agitation, and talkativeness, with alcohol odor on breath	• Alcohol or drug abuse	• Hidden GI bleeding • Psychiatric disorder; for example, mania • Subdural hematoma
Unilateral dilated pupil	• Neurologic disorder or injury	• Eye prosthesis • Previous eye injury
Multifocal premature ventricular contractions (PVCs)	• Severe heart disease	• Benign cardiac arrhythmia (of long standing) • Digitalis toxicity
Restlessness, belligerence, combativeness, bladder or bowel incontinence, poor hygienic habits, disheveled appearance	• Alcohol or drug abuse • Psychiatric disorder	• Brain lesion • Hypoxia
Hallucinations, delusions of grandeur, disorientation, or combativeness	• Psychiatric disorder; for example, psychosis • Alcohol or drug abuse	• Atypical reaction to drug overdose • Organic brain syndrome • Bacterial meningitis

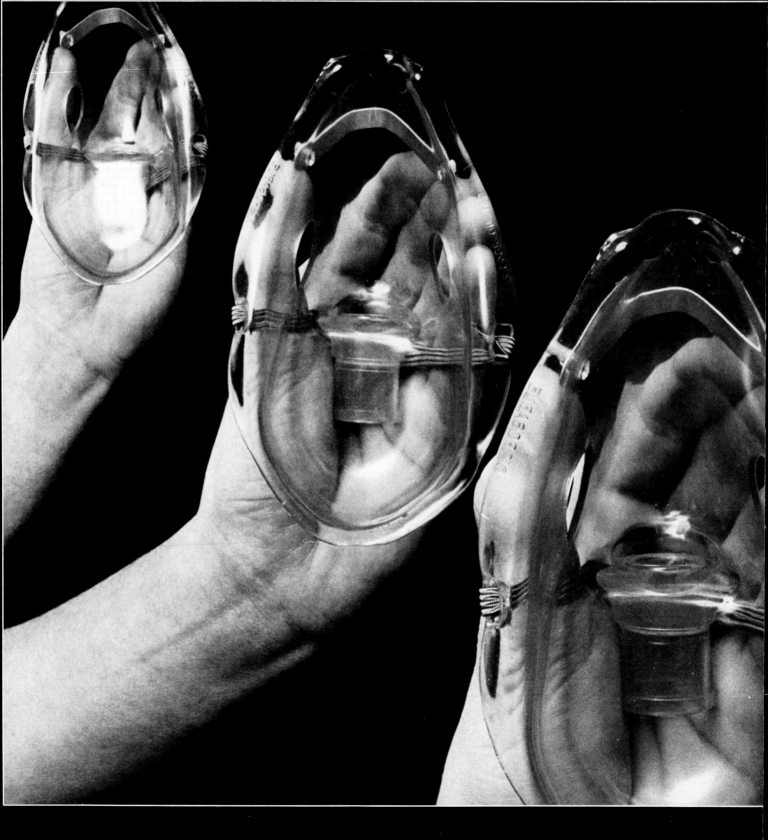

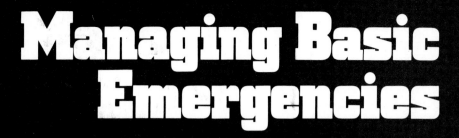

Managing Basic Emergencies

Airway management

Cardiopulmonary resuscitation

Hemorrhage

Burn care

Airway management

If a patient stops breathing suddenly, will you know what to do? For instance, can you clear an obstructed airway? Do you know how to give mouth-to-mouth respiration, mouth-to-nose respiration, or mouth-to-stoma respiration? Can you operate a hand-held resuscitator? Assist the doctor with a bedside tracheotomy? What precautions must you take with a patient who's had severe electrical shock?

If you're not sure what to do in these situations, study the following pages. They illustrate all the current techniques used in emergency airway management and explain how to avoid the more common pitfalls.

MINI-ASSESSMENT

Does your patient have an obstructed airway?

Suspect a partial or complete airway obstruction if your patient:
• begins clutching at his throat.
• can't speak but makes crowing noises (stridor).
• becomes pale or cyanotic.
• has exaggerated chest movements with retraction, especially during inspiration.
• begins wheezing suddenly.
• develops tachycardia.
• becomes restless, agitated, fearful.

Possible causes of airway obstruction include:
• aspirated food, or foreign bodies, such as teeth, dentures, or toys.
• anaphylaxis.
• unconsciousness, where the tongue falls back and blocks the airway.
• seizures.
• severe trauma to the face, neck, or upper chest.
• acute tracheal edema from smoke inhalation or from face and neck burns.

Remember: Absence of breathing doesn't always mean the patient has an airway obstruction. He may have:
• cardiopulmonary arrest.
• toxic reaction to an inhaled chemical, an anesthetic, or a drug.
• respiratory paralysis from a neuromuscular disease, like myasthenia gravis.
• head or spinal cord injury (cervical).
• oxygen toxicity.
Important: Always give a person with an airway obstruction *immediate* treatment. To find out how, read the following photostory.

How to clear an obstructed airway

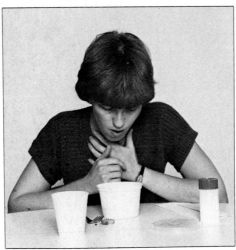

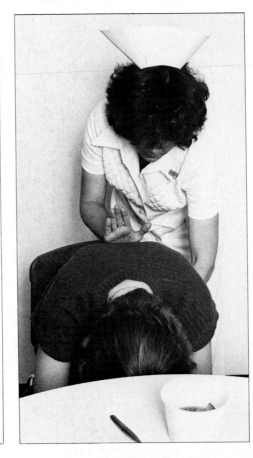

1 *Imagine yourself in this situation. You're eating lunch in the hospital cafeteria and you suddenly spot one of your co-workers choking on her food. How can you help?*

Quickly assess the problem. Does she have an airway obstruction? Be ready to intervene if she can't relieve the obstruction with forceful coughing.

Suppose her coughing seems weak or ineffective. Or she clutches her throat, makes crowing noises (stridor), or becomes cyanotic. Suspect a complete airway obstruction, and act quickly to remove it. If you don't, she'll suffer irreversible brain damage in 3 to 5 minutes.

Use one of the following techniques.

2 Is the patient standing or sitting down? Get behind her, as the nurse has positioned herself in this photo. Using one hand to support the patient's chest, bend her forward until her head is lower than her shoulders. Then, with the heel of your other hand, deliver four sharp blows over her spine, between the scapulae.

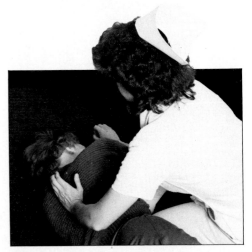

3 Is the patient lying down? Kneel next to her, and roll her onto her side, facing you. Then, brace your thigh against her chest and deliver four sharp blows to her back, as already described.

4 *Remember:* If your patient's a small child, place him over your knees, as shown here. Make sure his head is down, and he's bent at the waist. Support him with one hand, as the nurse is doing in this photo. With the heel of your other hand, deliver four back blows, as described earlier. *Note:* Is your patient an infant? Invert him over one arm to perform this procedure.

6 Suppose your patient's on the floor, and you can't lift her. Position her on her back, and turn her head to one side. Kneel astride her or alongside her hips, as shown here. Now, place your hands, one on top of the other, directly over her epigastrium. With the heel of your bottom hand, press upward with a quick thrust, to clear the airway.

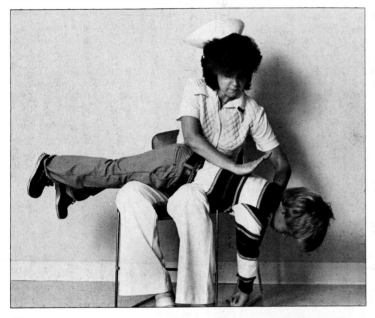

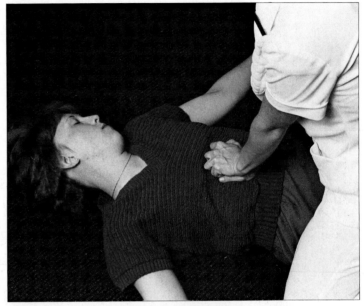

5 In some cases, the abdominal thrust may prove the best way to clear an obstructed airway. When done correctly, it can force enough air through the patient's airway to dislodge an obstruction.
 Here's how to perform the abdominal thrust. Stand behind her, as shown here, and wrap your arms around her waist. With one hand, make a fist and place the thumb side against the patient's epigastrium. Keep your fist above the patient's navel but below her xiphoid process. Then, grasp your fist with your other hand and press upward with a quick thrust. Repeat, if necessary.

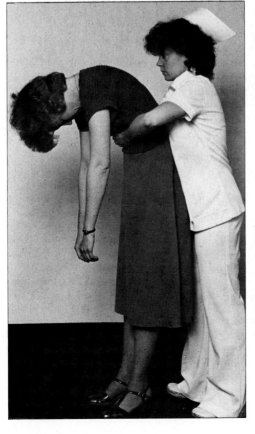

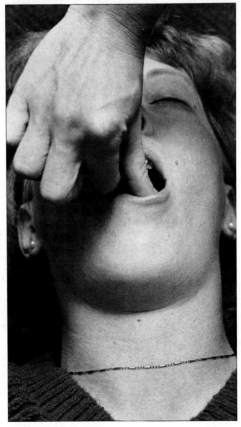

7 What if your patient's unconscious and you suspect an airway obstruction? Try removing the obstruction with your finger. Here's how:
 Immediately open her mouth, using the crossed-finger technique. To do this correctly, place your thumb on the patient's lower teeth and your index finger on her upper teeth, as shown here. Then, force her jaw downward with your thumb and upward with your index finger.
 ☎ *Nursing tip:* If your patient has dentures, remove them at once so they don't slip out of place and further obstruct her airway.

Airway management

How to clear an obstructed airway continued

8 Now, insert the index finger of your other hand deep inside the patient's throat. With a hooking motion, try to dislodge the foreign body and lift it out. Take care not to force the object deeper into her airway.

Note: Never attempt to remove an obstruction with your fingers if your patient's having a seizure.

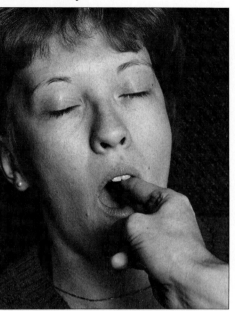
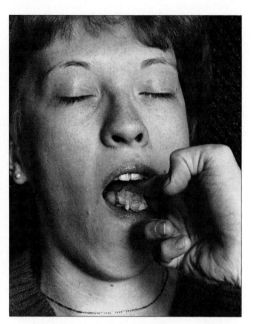

9 Did you remove the obstruction? Then, with two fingers, use a sweeping motion to clear the patient's mouth of any remaining vomitus, mucus, or blood. Once you've cleared her airway, restore breathing with artificial respiration, if necessary (see page 22).

Note: If you can't remove the obstruction using the above method, try back blows and abdominal thrusts.

Nurses' guide to pharyngeal airways

An oral or a nasal pharyngeal airway will maintain an air passage to the patient's posterior pharynx. For instructions on how to insert pharyngeal airways, read the following chart. For detailed, comprehensive instructions on inserting, cleaning, and removing pharyngeal airways, refer to the NURSING PHOTOBOOK *Providing Respiratory Care*, pages 28 to 31.

Type of airway	How to insert	Special nursing considerations
Oral pharyngeal	• First, open your patient's mouth, using the crossed-finger technique or a modified jaw thrust. Point the tip of the artificial airway toward the roof of your patient's mouth. • Now, gently advance the artificial airway until it slides into place. As you do, rotate it about 180°. • Is your patient an infant? Hold his tongue down with a tongue depressor. Then, guide the artificial airway over the back of his tongue until it slides into place. • Once the artificial airway's in place, secure it with two ½" adhesive strips. Use nonallergenic tape.	• If your patient gags as you're inserting the airway, do your best to reassure him. Then, hold the airway in place until he relaxes. • Once the airway's in place and taped securely, turn your patient's head to the side. Then, if he vomits, he won't aspirate the vomitus.
Nasal pharyngeal	• First, determine the correct tube length for your patient by measuring the distance from the tip of his nose to his earlobe. Mark this distance on the tube with tape. • Next, lubricate the tube with water or a water-soluble jelly. • With your fingers, gently push up the tip of your patient's nose, and insert the tube into his nostril. Stop when you reach the tape mark. • Now, ask the patient to exhale with his mouth closed. Do you feel air coming out of the tube? If you do, you've positioned the tube properly. • Finally, check the tube's position visually by using a tongue depressor to hold your patient's mouth open. Look for the tube's tip, which should be just behind the uvula. Secure the tube to your patient's cheek and nose with nonallergenic tape.	• You'll probably use this type of airway, rather than an oral pharyngeal airway, if your patient's had mouth trauma or surgery, or if he requires frequent suctioning. A nasal pharyngeal airway will help protect his oral mucosa from further injury. • If your patient's conscious, explain the procedure and why it's necessary, before you begin. Reassure him. • To ensure a snug fit, use a tube with an outside diameter slightly larger than your patient's nostril.

**How to give
mouth-to-mouth respiration**

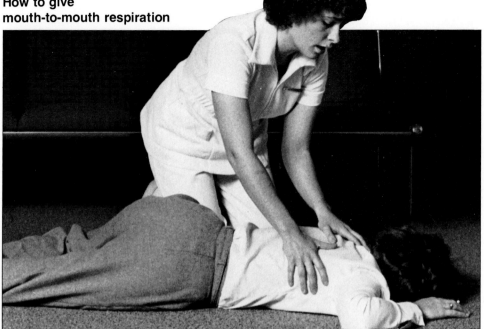

1 *You never know when an emergency will arise. For example, suppose you're on your way to another unit and discover a hospital visitor lying on the floor. Does she need artificial respiration? What about cardiopulmonary resuscitation (CPR)? Here's how to find out:*

First, determine if the person's unconscious by shaking her shoulder and shouting, "Can you hear me?" If she doesn't respond, call for help immediately. *Important:* Take care not to shake the patient too forcefully. Doing so could complicate any injuries she may have.

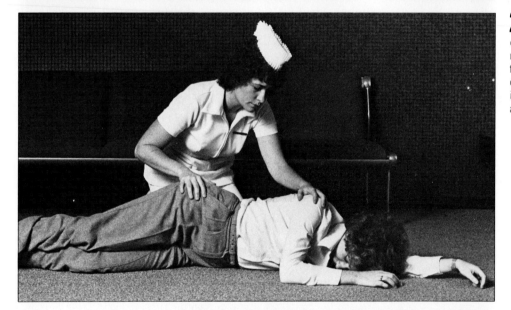

2 If the patient's lying face down or on her side, roll her on her back so you can give whatever emergency care she needs. Don't twist her body as you reposition it. Instead, roll it as a unit. Be especially careful if you suspect she has a neck injury; make sure her spine stays perfectly aligned.

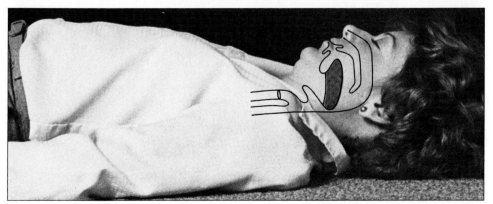

3 Now, study this picture. As you can see, when an unconscious patient's lying on her back, her lower jaw muscles relax, allowing her tongue to fall back and occlude her airway.

To correct this, you may use the head-tilt maneuver. To do this properly, hyperextend her neck by placing one hand beneath it and the other hand on her forehead.

Airway management

How to give mouth-to-mouth respiration continued

4 Now, lift the patient's neck with one hand and press down on her forehead with the other. As you can see in this illustration, this maneuver raises her tongue from the back of her throat and opens the airway.

Caution: Never hyperextend a patient's neck in this way if you suspect she has a spinal injury. Instead, use the modified jaw thrust, as described on page 23.

Nursing tip: Does your patient have dentures? Leave them in place. They'll help you get a better seal if you have to give mouth-to-mouth respiration. However, if the dentures are loose-fitting, remove them immediately.

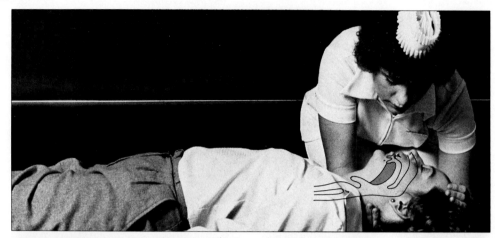

5 Now, check to see if your patient's breathing by placing your ear over her mouth and nose and observing her chest and abdomen. Listen and feel for air escaping during exhalation. Watch her chest to see if it rises and falls.

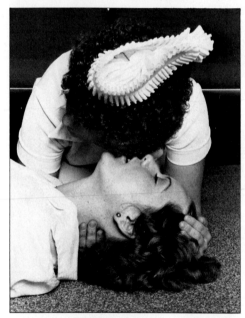

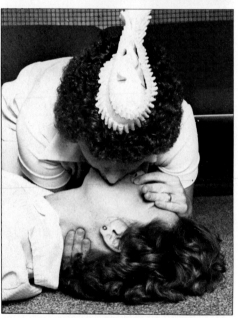

6 Occasionally, hyperextending the patient's neck isn't enough to lift her tongue and open her airway. If it isn't, try supporting her lower jaw by lifting her chin. To do this correctly, place your fingers under the bony—not soft—part of her lower jaw and bring her chin forward, as shown here. Use your thumb to lightly depress your patient's lower lip. *Never* use your thumb to lift her chin.

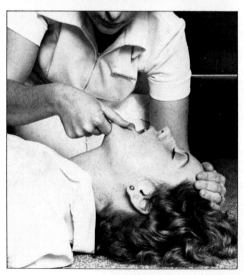

7 By this time, your patient should have an open airway, which may be enough to restore her breathing. If you notice that she's trying to breathe but you still don't feel or hear air passing through her airway, check again for an obstruction.

Now, consider this possibility. Suppose your patient's still not breathing, even after you've opened her airway. Begin artificial respiration immediately.

To do this properly, use the hand you've placed on her forehead to pinch her nostrils closed. Keep her neck hyperextended with your other hand. Now, take a deep breath, open your mouth very wide and place it around the outside of your patient's mouth. Make a tight seal. Then, quickly blow four full breaths into her lungs, without allowing time for them to deflate between breaths.

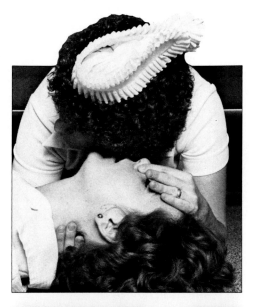

8 Now, turn your head so your cheek is close to the patient's mouth. Listen and feel for signs of restored breathing. Watch her chest to see if it rises and falls. If your first efforts to resuscitate the patient are unsuccessful, try again. Make sure your mouth is open wide enough to get a tight seal.

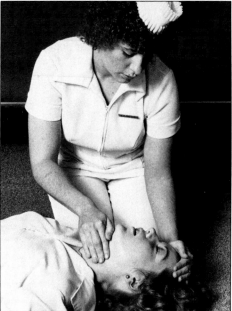

9 Now, feel for the patient's carotid pulse. To locate the carotid artery, first place your fingers on the patient's larynx. Then, slide them laterally into the groove between her trachea and the muscles on the side of her neck. Don't press the carotid artery too hard or you may cause a cardiac arrhythmia.

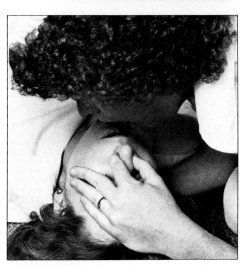

10 Suppose you can feel the patient's carotid pulse, but she's still not breathing. Deliver one breath every 5 seconds, as described in step 7. Recheck the carotid pulse after every 12 breaths to make sure it's still present. If it isn't, your patient's heart has stopped beating. Start cardiopulmonary resuscitation (CPR) immediately. For full details on how to give CPR correctly, see pages 27 through 30.

Important: Never give CPR to a patient whose heart is still beating. To avoid this mistake, be sure to check carefully for a carotid pulse.

How to do a modified jaw thrust

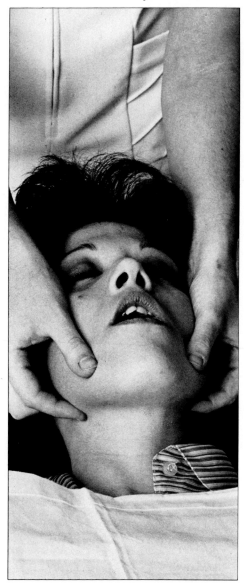

Hyperextending a patient's neck isn't the only way to open her airway. Nor is it the correct way if your patient has a spinal injury. Instead, use the modified jaw thrust shown in this photo. Here's how to do it:

First, stand just behind your patient, as the nurse is doing here. Next, grasp the angles of her lower jaw, directly in front of her earlobes. Make sure your thumbs rest on the bony area of the jaw. If you grasp the jaw's soft tissue, you may add to the obstruction of the airway.

Now, lift her lower jaw upward, so that it juts forward. Done correctly, the modified jaw thrust will open the patient's airway without hyperextending her neck. If you must also give her mouth-to-mouth respiration, retract her lower lip with your thumbs.

Airway management

When an infant needs artificial respiration

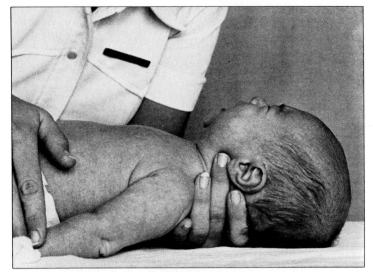 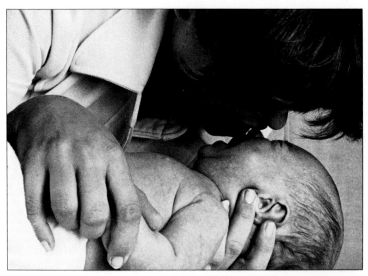

1 *What if an infant stops breathing and needs artificial respiration? Do you know how to proceed? First, check for an airway obstruction and remove it, if possible. If no obstruction's present and the infant still isn't breathing, follow the usual mouth-to-mouth procedure, with these special guidelines:*

Place one hand or a folded towel underneath the infant's shoulders to hyperextend his neck properly. Never hyperextend an infant's neck as much as you would an adult's. Doing so could block the infant's airway. In some cases, it may damage his spinal cord.

2 Now, place your mouth over the infant's nose and mouth. Get a tight seal. Then, deliver four quick breaths like puffs of air. Never breathe forcefully into an infant's lungs. Doing so could overinflate them.

Watch for signs of gastric distention, which may occur if air enters the infant's stomach. To relieve marked distention, turn the infant on his side and gently apply pressure to his abdomen. Then, if he vomits, he won't aspirate the vomitus.

Giving mouth-to-nose respiration

What do you do when a patient with a crushed jaw needs artificial respiration? Since you can't give her mouth-to-mouth respiration, try the mouth-to-nose method. (You may also want to use this method when you can't get a tight seal on a patient who's toothless.)

To give mouth-to-nose respiration properly, follow these steps: First, open the patient's airway by hyperextending her neck or using the modified jaw thrust (if she also has spinal injuries). Make sure her mouth is tightly closed by pressing your thumb lightly against her lips.

Now, place your open mouth over her nose, with your cheek against her lips. Take care to get a tight seal; then give artificial respiration in the usual way.

📞 *Nursing tip:* If no air escapes from the patient's nose during exhalation, open her mouth. Her soft palate may be blocking her nasal passages. Don't forget to close her mouth before you resume ventilations.

One other important point: Check the patient's carotid pulse after the first four breaths; then again after every twelve breaths. If it's absent, begin cardiopulmonary resuscitation (CPR) immediately.

Giving mouth-to-stoma respiration

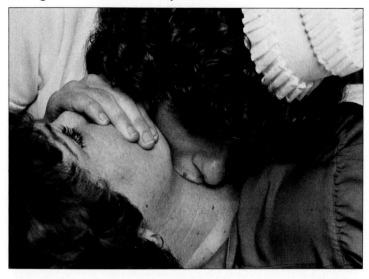

When a laryngectomee needs artificial respiration, use the mouth-to-stoma method. Why? Because most of the air you breathe into her mouth or nose won't reach her lungs. To perform mouth-to-stoma respiration correctly, follow these instructions:

First, make sure the patient is lying flat on her back. Don't hyperextend her neck or let her head turn to either side because this could alter the shape of her stoma, blocking her airway. When the patient's properly positioned, cover her mouth and nose with your hand, as the nurse is doing here.

Now, seal your mouth over her stoma and deliver four full breaths in rapid succession. Don't wait for her lungs to deflate between breaths. Watch her chest closely to see if it rises and falls.

Remove your mouth from her stoma, and use your fingers to feel for a carotid pulse. If a pulse is present, continue to deliver breaths (one every 5 seconds) until breathing's restored. If no pulse is present, start cardiopulmonary resuscitation (CPR) immediately. For full details on how to do this, see pages 27 through 30. *Important:* Always check for a carotid pulse after every 12 breaths. Remember, your patient's heart could stop beating at any time.

How to use a hand-held resuscitator

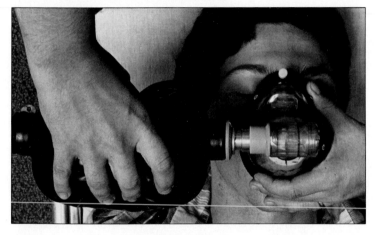

Giving emergency mouth-to-mouth respiration in a hospital or clinic? Be prepared for someone to relieve you with a hand-held resuscitator. Here's how to use one:

First, attach the mask to the bag, and connect the resuscitator to the oxygen source. Then, hyperextend the patient's neck and place the mask over his face. *Important:* Make sure the apex of the triangle is over the bridge of his nose and the base is between his lower lip and chin. (Study this photo.)

Now, firmly hold the mask in place to create a tight seal. Compress the bag with your other hand. Or, if you prefer, compress it against your side, using your lower arm.

Watch to make sure the patient's chest wall rises and falls each time the bag is compressed. If it doesn't, you may not have a tightly sealed mask. Reposition your hands and try again.

For more details on how to use a hand-held resuscitator, see the NURSING PHOTOBOOK *Providing Respiratory Care.*

How to do a cricothyreotomy

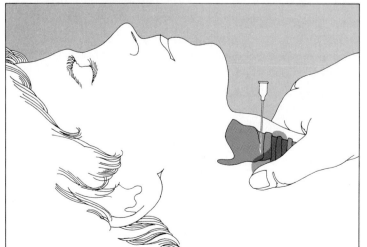

You're driving home late one night when the car in front of you skids off the road. Since you're the only health-care professional at the scene, you quickly assess the victim and find he's not breathing. You deliver artificial respiration without response, and all attempts to open his airway fail. To save his life, you'll have to perform an emergency cricothyreotomy.

Here's how: First, gently grasp the victim's trachea. Then, slide your fingers downward, to locate his thyroid gland. You'll know you're at the outer borders of the thyroid gland when the space between your fingers and thumb widens. Next, move your index finger across the center of the gland, over the anterior edge of the cricoid ring. Now, cut or stab the victim's cricothyroid membrane, just below the cricoid ring. Insert something hollow to keep the airway open; for example, a pen with the cartridge removed or a drinking straw.

Study this illustration to better understand where to make a cricoid stab. *Important:* You'd *never* attempt a cricothyreotomy unless it were an *extreme* emergency, like the situation described above. When the procedure's done in a hospital—in a life-or-death situation—the doctor or nurse may use a 14G needle, as shown here.

Airway management

The bedside tracheotomy: Your role

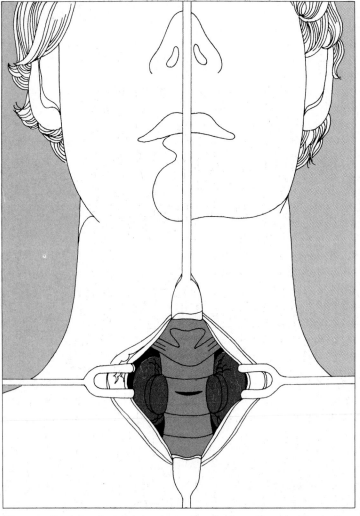

If your patient needs a tracheotomy, the doctor will probably do the procedure in the OR. However, in an extreme emergency, he may need to perform a tracheotomy at the patient's bedside. What's your role during such a procedure? Follow these instructions:

First, quickly reassure the patient, and explain what to expect. As you do, assemble the necessary equipment: trach tray, sterile gloves (several pairs), Betadine, sterile water, 3-0 and 4-0 size silk sutures, 5 cc syringe, 22G needle, and a local anesthetic. In addition, gather suctioning equipment (including sterile saline solution) and equipment for possible emergency resuscitation.

Now, make sure the working area is well lighted. Remove the bed's headboard so you have enough room to administer oxygen and use a hand-held resuscitator, if necessary.

When the doctor's ready to make the incision but not before, prepare the patient by placing him flat on his back. Put a small, rolled towel under his shoulders to hyperextend his neck and properly align his mouth and trachea.

Study this illustration to see where the doctor will make the incision for a tracheotomy. Note how its position differs from that of the cricoid stab, illustrated on page 25.

When the doctor's completed the procedure, document it in your nurses' notes. Continue to observe the patient closely for signs of edema or bleeding. If either develops, notify the doctor.

How to reinsert a trach tube

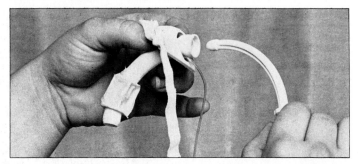

If your patient coughs out his trach tube, reinsert it at once. To do this properly, proceed as follows: Quickly reassure him, telling him what you're doing. Then, as you remove the inner cannula from the dislodged trach tube, *check to make sure the cuff's deflated.* Take the obturator that's usually on the bedside table or taped to the headboard, and insert it in the trach's outer cannula. Next, reinsert the trach tube (with obturator) into the patient's stoma.

Hold the trach plate securely in place, and remove the obturator. Reinsert the inner cannula, and lock it in place, using a clockwise motion. Now, inflate the cuff, and secure the trach ties and bib around the trach plate. Auscultate the patient's lungs to make sure he's getting enough air. Document the entire episode in your notes. (For complete details on this procedure, read the NURSING PHOTOBOOK *Providing Respiratory Care.*)

When the patient has an esophageal obturator airway

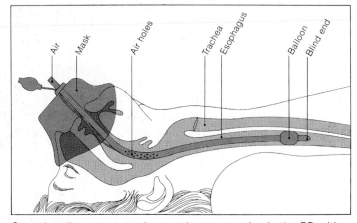

Occasionally, an unconscious patient may arrive in the ED with an esophageal obturator airway (EOA) in place. Such an airway is usually inserted by an emergency medical technician, who isn't permitted to intubate with an endotracheal tube. Do you know how to manage a patient with an EOA? These guidelines will help.

First, study the illustration above to see how an EOA works. Notice how this special airway is inserted into the patient's esophagus, rather than his trachea. The cuffed end of the tube is closed so that administered air or oxygen can't pass through it. Instead, the air or oxygen passes through the tube's special air holes into the patient's trachea. The inflated cuff keeps the airway in place and prevents any regurgitated stomach contents from reaching the trachea.

Never remove an EOA until the doctor's found another way to secure a patent airway. Deflate the cuff before you remove it.

Cardiopulmonary resuscitation

Giving CPR to adults

When was the last time you administered cardiopulmonary resuscitation (CPR)? If it's been awhile, you probably need to review the basic technique. Whether you work in a hospital or a clinic, you must be prepared to perform this lifesaving procedure correctly and without hesitation.

Refresh your CPR skills by studying the following pages. Review how to:
* give CPR to an adult or an infant.
* give CPR by yourself or with another person.
* move the patient while you're giving CPR.
* use the defibrillator.

You'll also find out when and how to give a precordial thump. *Important:* Never give CPR without first being trained by a certified instructor. Use the photostories included here only to review the proper technique.

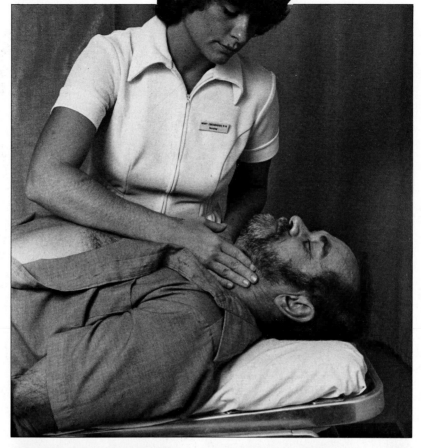

1 *You're on duty in the emergency department. Suddenly, the patient you're caring for stops breathing. When you assess his condition, you discover he has no carotid pulse. He needs immediate cardiopulmonary resuscitation (CPR), or irreversible brain damage will occur in 3 to 5 minutes.*

Do you know how to give CPR correctly? Get the training you need from a qualified instructor. Then, study this photostory to review the basic technique.

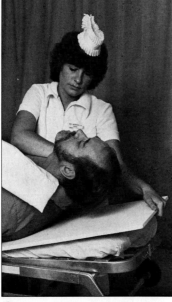

2 First, make sure your patient's lying on a firm surface. If he's on a bed or a stretcher, put a CPR board under him.

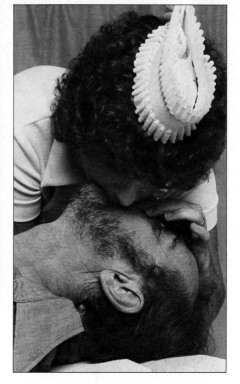

3 Now, kneel or stand beside the patient so you can begin CPR. Is your patient on a stretcher like the one shown here? Stand on a stool so you can position yourself correctly for chest compressions.

Open the patient's airway by hyperextending his neck or using one of the methods described on pages 18 to 20 and 23. Then, ventilate his lungs with four quick, full breaths before you proceed further.

Cardiopulmonary resuscitation

Giving CPR to adults continued

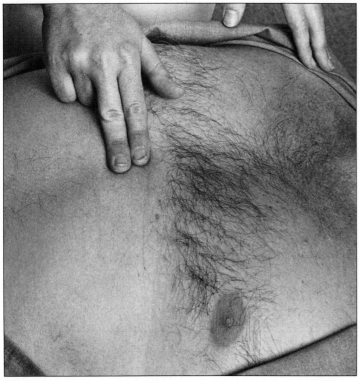

4 Now, you're ready to position your hands for chest compressions. Begin by first locating the xiphoid process, which is at the lower end of the patient's sternum. Measure 1½" to 2" (3.8 to 5 cm)—or approximately two finger-widths—up from this point. You'll give chest compressions *in this area*.

Important: Never give chest compressions directly *over* the patient's xiphoid process. Doing so may lacerate his liver.

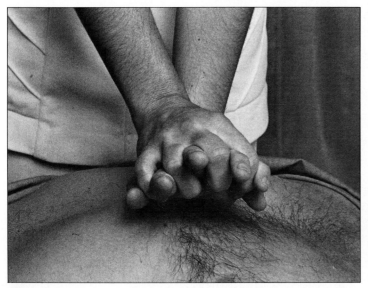

5 Now, place one hand on top of the other, as the nurse in this photo is doing. Interlock your fingers so you're sure of keeping them off the chest wall.

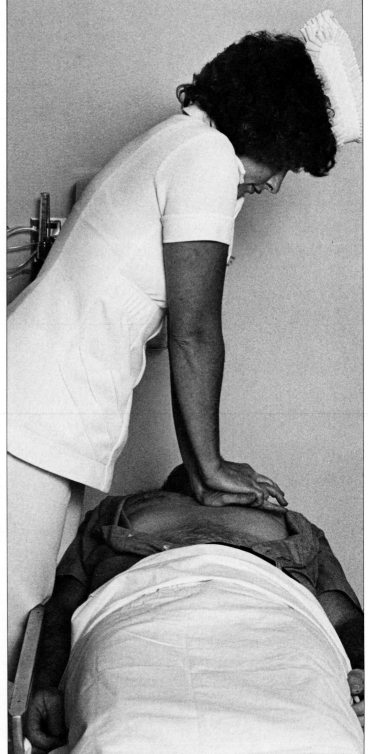

6 Lean forward so that your shoulders are directly over the patient's sternum and your arms are at a 90° angle to his chest. Keep your arms straight to minimize fatigue and to use your weight effectively.

7 With the heel of your hand, exert pressure downward, depressing the patient's sternum 1½" to 2" (3.8 to 5 cm). This pressure squeezes the heart between the sternum and the vertebral column and forces blood from the heart's chambers.

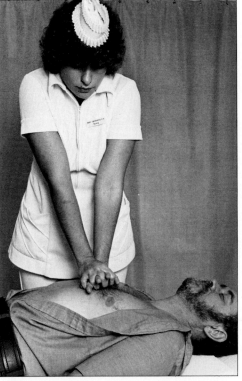

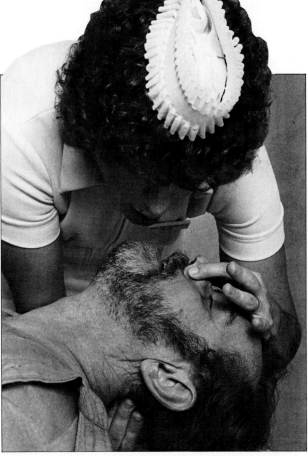

8 After each chest compression, release *all pressure* to allow the sternum to return to its normal position. This action will permit the heart's chambers to refill.

Important: Don't remove your hands from the patient's chest when you release pressure on his sternum. Doing so may cause you to lose correct hand placement.

Perform this compression/relaxation sequence at a rate of 80 per minute. Work smoothly and rhythmically, making sure compression and relaxation times are equal. To maintain this rhythm, count aloud: "One- and, two- and, three- and," and so on.

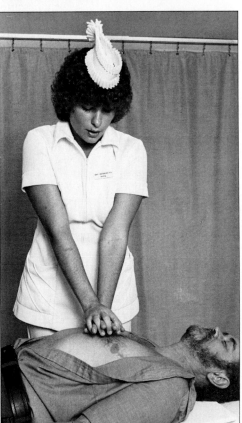

9 As you may know, for CPR to be effective, your patient must also receive artificial respiration along with chest compressions. If you're working alone, accomplish this by giving the patient two quick lung inflations after every fifteen chest compressions. Deliver these breaths in rapid succession, without allowing the patient to exhale fully between breaths.

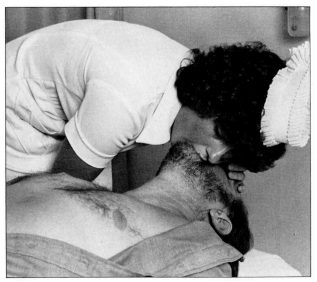

10 While you're inflating the patient's lungs, watch his chest to see if it rises and falls. After performing CPR for 1 minute, check his carotid pulse. If it's still absent, continue CPR until someone relieves you.

Cardiopulmonary resuscitation

How to give CPR to an adult continued

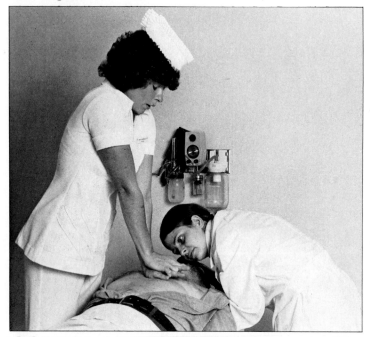

11 If another nurse or a trained person can help you give CPR, one should inflate the patient's lungs while the other applies chest compressions. You can position yourselves on the same side of the patient, but if CPR must continue for an extended period, you'll be better off working on opposite sides, as shown here.

For two-person CPR, give chest compressions at a rate of 60 per minute, with one lung inflation after every five chest compressions.

For best results, the person giving compressions should count aloud, "one-one thousand, two-one thousand, three-one thousand," and so on.

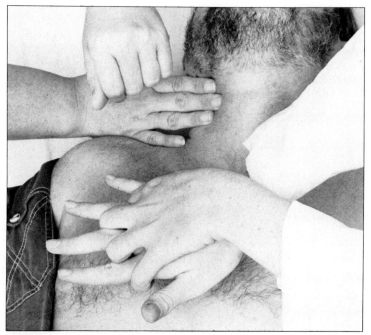

12 If the person giving chest compressions tires and needs to switch positions, she notifies her helper by saying (in rhythm), "Change one-thousand, two-one thousand, three-one thousand, four-one thousand, five-one thousand." Then, the helper giving lung inflations delivers one breath and moves into position for chest compressions. Now the person giving chest compressions completes the compression sequence, moves next to the patient's head and checks his carotid pulse for 5 seconds, *but no longer.* If no carotid pulse is felt, she delivers a breath and tells the helper giving chest compressions, "continue CPR." But if she feels a carotid pulse she'll say, "there's a pulse" and continue to give artificial respirations.

Giving CPR to an infant or child

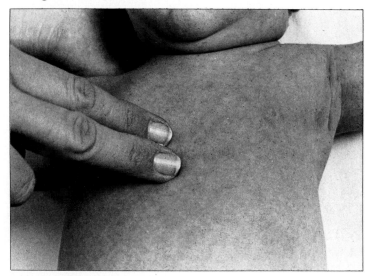

On page 24 we showed you how to give artificial respiration to an infant or a child. Here's what to do if you're also giving him CPR:

For infants, you'll need to deliver 100 chest compressions per minute. Is your patient a child? Deliver 80 chest compressions per minute, using only the heel of *one* hand to compress his sternum 1″ to 1½″ (2.5 to 3.8 cm). With an infant, use just the tips of your index and middle fingers to compress his sternum ½″ to 1″ (1.3 to 2.5 cm), as shown in this photo. More forceful compressions could injure the infant's or child's liver.

What's on the crash cart?

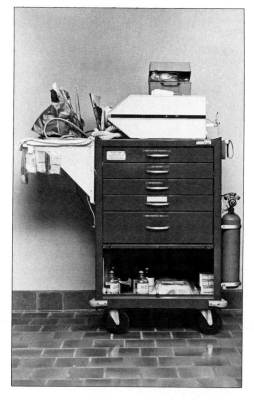

When a code's called in your unit and the code team arrives with a crash cart, will you be prepared to help effectively? For example, do you know what's included on a hospital crash cart? You should. When seconds count, you must be able to find what you need without delay.

Take the time to carefully examine one of your unit's crash carts. Go over its equipment, item by item, until you know what everything's for and where to find it.

Although crash carts vary from hospital to hospital, a typical cart includes the following equipment: defibrillator with paddles, electrode jelly, saline pads, and a CPR board; oxygen cylinder (D size) with O_2 tubing and masks; a suction machine with suction catheters; a hand-held resuscitator; a laryngoscope tray with blades and endotracheal tubes; assorted oral and nasal airways, stylet, and padded tongue blades; a cutdown tray; assorted I.V. solutions, catheters and needles, additive labels, armboard, and tourniquets; an arterial blood sampling kit, assorted syringes and needles, including intracardiac and spinal needles; a trach tray; a nasogastric tube with bulb syringe; a CVP manometer; disposable scalpels; hemostats; 4" x 4" and 2" x 2" sterile gauze pads; adhesive tape; alcohol swabs; assorted sutures; and sterile gloves.

Drugs usually found on a crash cart include: atropine sulfate, bretylium tosylate (Bretylol), calcium chloride, calcium gluconate*, deslanoside (Cedilanid*), dextrose 50%, diazepam (Valium*), diazoxide (Hyperstat*), digoxin*, dopamine HCl (Intropin*), epinephrine HCl, furosemide (Lasix*), isoproterenol HCl (Isuprel*), levarterenol (Levophed*), lidocaine HCl (Xylocaine*), mannitol*, metaraminol bitartrate (Aramine*), methylprednisolone sodium succinate (Solu-Medrol*), naloxone HCl (Narcan*), ouabain, phenytoin sodium (Dilantin*), procainamide HCl (Pronestyl*), propranolol HCl (Inderal*), quinidine*, and sodium bicarbonate*. *Know these drugs' actions and side effects.*

Important: To ensure cleanliness, keep your unit's crash cart covered when not in use. Assign someone to check the cart daily (and after each code) to restock supplies and to test the defibrillator. Also, check the expiration dates on drugs, and trach and cutdown trays. Replace them with new supplies, if necessary.

*Available in the United States and in Canada.

How to give a precordial thump

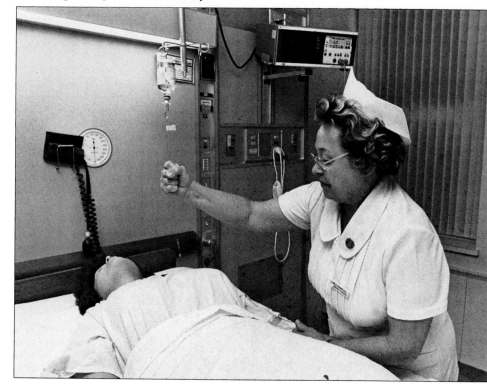

You're caring for 35-year-old Mrs. James, who's 2 hours postop a bowel resection. Suddenly, her cardiac monitor alarm sounds, indicating she's suffered cardiac arrest. Do you know what to do?

Before you begin CPR, try a precordial thump to restore her heartbeat. You may attempt a precordial thump within 1 minute after you witness a monitored arrest. Never try this maneuver under any other circumstance.

Here's how you do it: Using the fleshy portion of your fist, deliver a sharp blow to the patient's midsternum. Then, immediately check the cardiac monitor for signs of a restored heartbeat. (To double-check, feel the patient's neck for a carotid pulse.) If no pulse is present, begin CPR immediately, using the guidelines on pages 27 to 30. Don't waste precious time giving repeated blows.

Important: Never try a precordial thump on an infant or child before you begin CPR. Such a blow could damage undeveloped ribs or cause internal bleeding.

Cardiopulmonary resuscitation

How to use a defibrillator

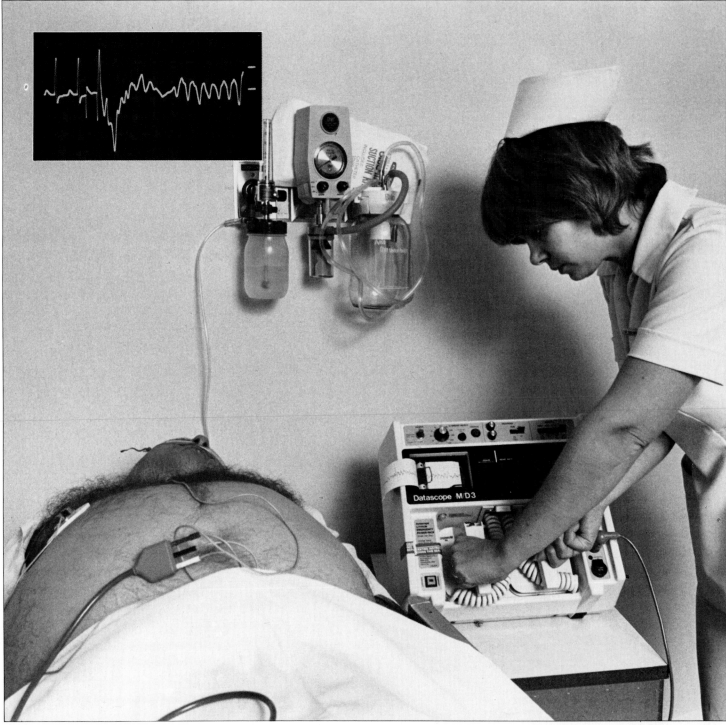

1 *Let's suppose you're working the night shift in the ED and Mr. Wills, a 58-year-old cabdriver, has just arrived complaining of severe epigastric pain. As you take his health history, he tells you he had a myocardial infarction (MI) 3 years ago. You immediately connect him to a cardiac* monitor, take his vital signs, and reassure him. Suddenly, the cardiac monitor shows his heart's in ventricular fibrillation (see inset). You call for help at once.

What next? Because the doctor's not available, you realize that you will have to defibrillate Mr. Wills. As you begin this emergency procedure, another ED nurse arrives to assist. *Important:* You should *never* attempt to use a defibrillator unless you've been trained properly. This photo-story reviews the basics. Read it carefully and you'll find out all you need to know about operating a defibrillator.

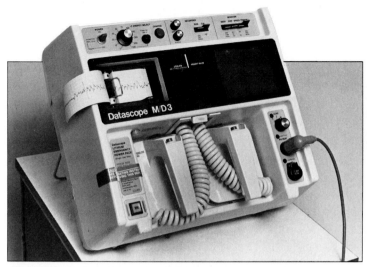

2 Depending on which type of defibrillator you're using, make sure the batteries are charged or that the electrical cord's plugged in. Also make sure the paddles are connected to the machine. Then, switch on the power.

Here, we're using the Datascope M/D3 Defibrillator System.® This portable, battery-operated machine has a built-in cardiac monitor, defibrillator, and cardiac-recording strip. Chest leads are attached to your patient to determine his cardiac activity. *Note:* Suppose your defibrillator doesn't have a built-in cardiac monitor. Use limb leads from an EKG machine.

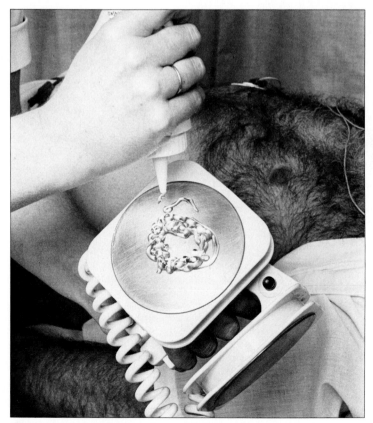

3 Now, quickly prepare the paddles so you can apply them to the patient's chest. To do this, you'll use a special electrode jelly that conducts electricity. 🖝 *Nursing tip:* Always keep a tube of jelly with the defibrillator.

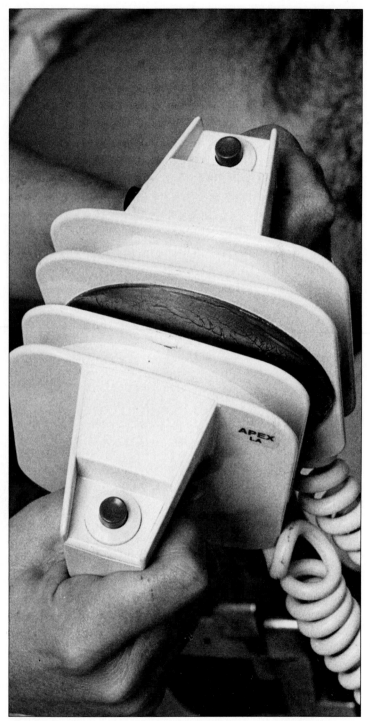

4 To reduce the risk of skin burns, put jelly on the paddles and coat the entire surface of each paddle by rubbing them against each other. But take care not to smear any jelly on yourself or the patient.

🖝 *Nursing tip:* Suppose you don't have any jelly on hand. You may use saline pads between the paddles and the patient's skin. However, never use alcohol pads for this purpose. Alcohol pads conduct electricity poorly and may catch fire.

Cardiopulmonary resuscitation

How to use a defibrillator continued

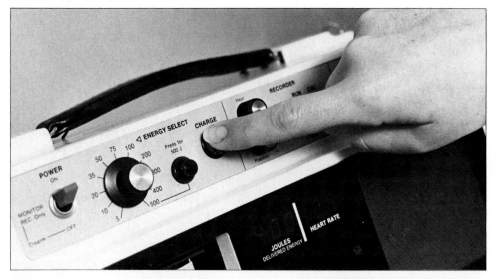

5 Set the control panel on the defibrillator so the machine will deliver the exact electrical charge the doctor's ordered. In most cases, an average adult patient will need 400 joules; a small adult or child will need 200 joules. *Note:* Your defibrillator may use watt-seconds instead of joules. In such a case, 400 watt-seconds are equal to 400 joules.

Now, charge the defibrillator by depressing the charge button until the gauge registers the prescribed number of joules or watt-seconds.

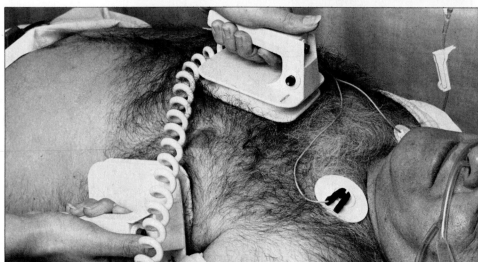

6 Place the paddles on the patient's chest, as shown here. Put one to the right of his sternum, on the second and third intercostal spaces, and the other near the heart's apex, along the left axillary line.

Not every machine is equipped with paddles like these, however. If the machine you're using has anterior/posterior paddles, position them as shown in the next illustration.

Important: Make sure both paddles are flat against the patient's skin. If they aren't, you may cause an electrical arc, which will burn both you and the patient. Dangerous arcing may also occur if the paddles are less than 2" (5 cm) apart.

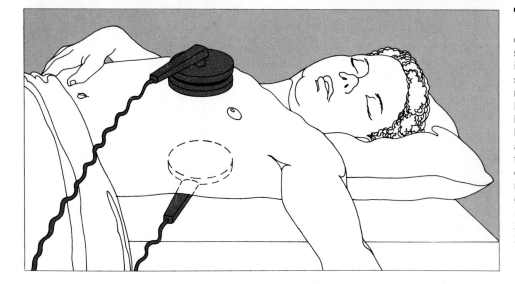

7 Suppose your patient is an infant or a small child. In this case, use a machine with anterior/posterior paddles. To position these paddles correctly, follow these instructions: First, turn the patient on his side. Now, place the posterior paddle beneath him, so it rests between his shoulder blades when he's lying flat on his back. Now, place the anterior paddle on his chest, between his left nipple and his sternum, as shown in this illustration. Charge the defibrillator for the prescribed amount of electricity. To calculate the number of joules needed for a small child or an infant, the doctor will probably use this formula (no matter which type of defibrillator is used): 2 joules per kg body weight, not to exceed 200 joules.

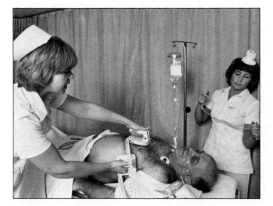

8 When the paddles are in place, tell everyone to stand clear of the patient and his bed. Make sure someone's turned off the oxygen (if it's in use). Check where you're standing to be sure you're on a *dry* floor. Now, look around to be certain no one's near the bed, and announce *loudly* that you're going to discharge the defibrillator. Then, simultaneously press the red discharge buttons on both handles.

After defibrillation, always examine your patient for possible skin burns. Treat them according to the doctor's orders. Document their size, appearance, and your care of them in your nurses' notes.

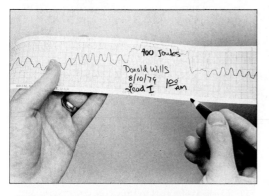

9 When you've administered the prescribed electrical charge, have someone record the date, time, lead, and prescribed joules or watt-seconds on the recording strip. Check for changes in heart rhythm. Start CPR, if needed.

After 1 minute, stop chest compressions, and check the patient's heart rhythm again. If the shock did not produce the desired change in rhythm, examine the leads to make sure they're still attached correctly. Change them, if necessary. Then, repeat defibrillation, if the doctor orders it. To do this, recharge the machine as instructed earlier, and follow safety precautions.

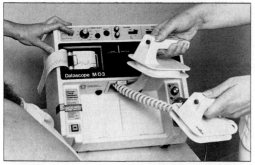

10 Suppose further defibrillation's unnecessary, but the machine's still charged. Separate the paddles by at least 4" (10 cm), and clear the charge by turning off the machine, as shown here, or by pressing the BLEED button, if your machine has one.

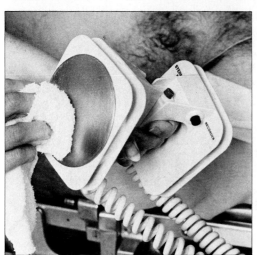

11 When you've completed the procedure, clean the defibrillator paddles with soap and water, taking care to remove all electrode jelly. Any jelly that remains will corrode the metal paddle heads, which can lead to skin burns from electrical arcs.

Now, get the defibrillator ready for immediate reuse. To do this, set the lead selector to the *LEAD II* position, and turn the sweep speed control to 25 mm per second. If the machine has a patient cable for monitoring heart rhythm, make sure it's connected to the machine. Restock the machine with electrode jelly and saline pads, if necessary.

Important: Assign someone in your unit to check the defibrillator at the beginning of each shift. Then, if the machine's not working properly, it can be replaced immediately.

AT THE SCENE

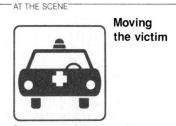

Moving the victim

Suppose you're giving CPR to a man who's had a cardiac arrest in your church one Sunday. Do you know how to move him properly when the emergency medical technicians (EMTs) arrive with the ambulance? If you're not sure, check these guidelines:

• Don't attempt to move the patient until everyone's ready. Keep in mind that you must never interrupt CPR for more than 5 seconds unless you're moving the patient up or down a stairway.

• Position the litter close to the patient. Now, stop giving CPR momentarily while you logroll the patient on his side. Quickly slide a CPR board underneath him. Resume CPR as soon as the EMTs have lifted him on the litter.

Important: Does the patient have a possible spinal cord injury? Make sure he has a cervical collar in place before you move him.

• Unless you're instructed otherwise, continue to give CPR as the patient's slowly wheeled to the ambulance. If you approach a stairway, prepare to stop CPR on a given signal. Move the patient up or down the stairway quickly. Then resume CPR again when the patient's on the next level. On stairways, *never* discontinue CPR for more than 15 seconds.

• If you've been asked to accompany the patient to the hospital, continue to give him CPR for as long as necessary in the ambulance. As you do, take special care to brace yourself properly while the vehicle's in motion.

Hemorrhage

As you know, vascular emergencies challenge you to work swiftly and competently. Any patient who's hemorrhaging internally, externally, or both needs your immediate care to save his life. Are you skilled enough to give it? The next several pages will help you cope effectively in such a situation. Read these pages to find out:

- when and how to apply pressure to a bleeding wound.
- how to remove a MAST suit.
- how to recognize and treat hypovolemic shock.

Using direct pressure to control bleeding

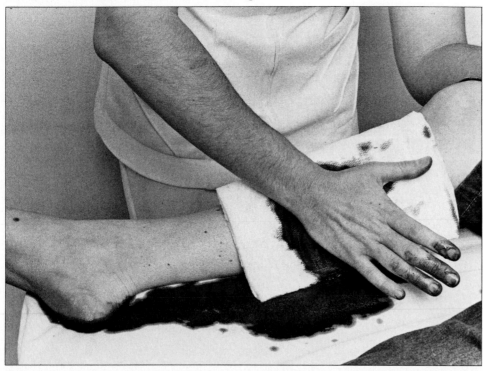

1 *Is your patient bleeding from an open wound? Do your best to control it by applying direct pressure. Always try direct pressure before you try anything else. Depending on the wound, you can use any of these three methods: hand pressure (over a sterile dressing, if possible), a pressure bandage, or a plastic air splint. If these methods fail to control the bleeding quickly, try using the pressure point method described on page 38.*

Here's how to apply hand pressure. First, place a thick, sterile dressing directly over the bleeding wound. Then, apply direct pressure with the heel of your hand, as shown here. Check the area every 5 to 10 minutes to see if the bleeding's stopped. If it hasn't, put another dressing *on top of the saturated one* and resume pressure. In such a case, never remove the saturated dressing to replace it with a clean one.

Suppose you don't have a sterile dressing handy. Use a clean cloth instead.

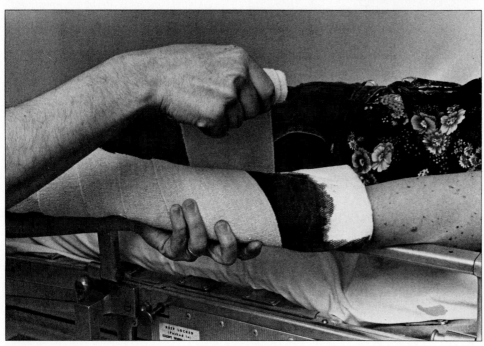

2 Does your patient have massive bleeding from an arm or leg wound? Apply a pressure bandage to maintain direct pressure over a long period. To do this, first place a thick, sterile dressing directly on top of the wound. Then, wrap the affected area with an elastic bandage, starting from the end of the extremity and moving toward the heart. To ensure even pressure, wrap the bandage smoothly and evenly, as shown here. Secure it with metal fasteners or adhesive tape.

4 Suppose your patient's been in a car accident and has chest injuries, as well as a severely bleeding leg wound. In such a case, his chest injuries may need attention first. So, while the doctor inserts a chest tube, he may want you to put a plastic air splint on the patient's leg. Here's how:

First, place a thick, sterile dressing directly on the affected area. Then, slip the splint over the dressing and inflate it.

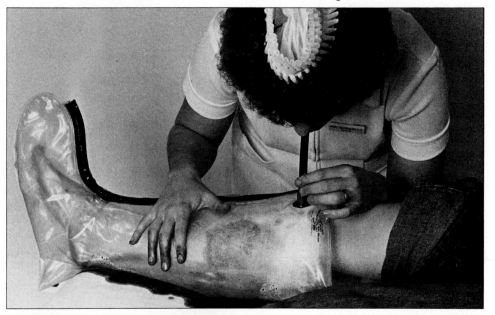

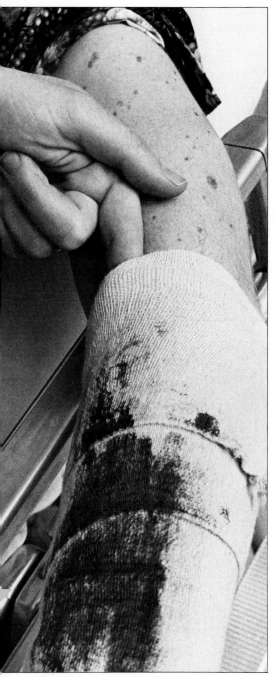

3 When you've secured the bandage, check your patient's circulation. If he complains of numbness, or has cool or mottled skin, blanched nailbeds, or no pulse in this arm or leg, you've probably wrapped the bandage too tightly. Remove it at once and reapply.

 Nursing tip: Here's an easy way to tell if you've applied the bandage correctly. Make sure you can easily slip your finger between the bandage and the patient's skin.

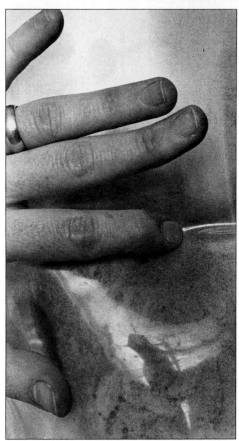

5 Keep in mind that a plastic air splint exerts circumferential pressure. If you overinflate it, you'll impede the patient's limb circulation. So, once the splint's applied, check his circulation, as explained in step 3. To test air pressure within the inflated splint, press down on it with your fingers. If the air pressure's correct, you should be able to indent the plastic about ½" (1.3 cm).

Always check the splinted arm or leg every 15 minutes to see if the bleeding's decreased or stopped. However, don't remove the splint each time. Instead, look through the clear plastic to observe the drainage.

Never remove the splint without a doctor's supervision, even though you applied it yourself. To remove the splint, first take the patient's blood pressure. Then, open the splint air valve, and release the air gradually at 5-minute intervals. Continue ongoing checks of the patient's blood pressure to make sure it remains stable. If it falls, the doctor may want you to reinflate the splint.

Hemorrhage

Using pressure points to control bleeding

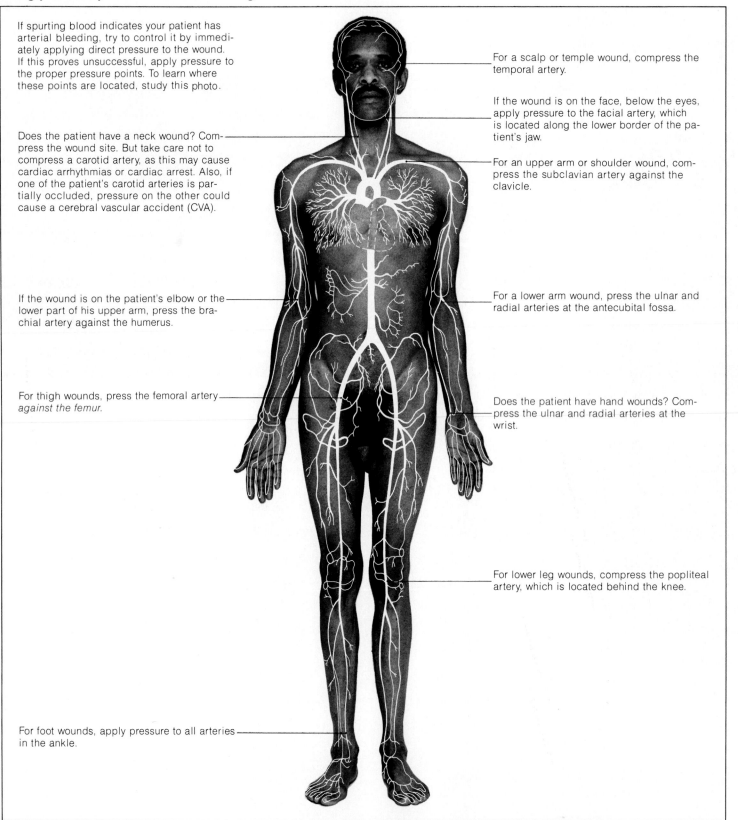

If spurting blood indicates your patient has arterial bleeding, try to control it by immediately applying direct pressure to the wound. If this proves unsuccessful, apply pressure to the proper pressure points. To learn where these points are located, study this photo.

Does the patient have a neck wound? Compress the wound site. But take care not to compress a carotid artery, as this may cause cardiac arrhythmias or cardiac arrest. Also, if one of the patient's carotid arteries is partially occluded, pressure on the other could cause a cerebral vascular accident (CVA).

If the wound is on the patient's elbow or the lower part of his upper arm, press the brachial artery against the humerus.

For thigh wounds, press the femoral artery *against the femur.*

For foot wounds, apply pressure to all arteries in the ankle.

For a scalp or temple wound, compress the temporal artery.

If the wound is on the face, below the eyes, apply pressure to the facial artery, which is located along the lower border of the patient's jaw.

For an upper arm or shoulder wound, compress the subclavian artery against the clavicle.

For a lower arm wound, press the ulnar and radial arteries at the antecubital fossa.

Does the patient have hand wounds? Compress the ulnar and radial arteries at the wrist.

For lower leg wounds, compress the popliteal artery, which is located behind the knee.

Internal bleeding: What's your role?

How can you tell if your patient's bleeding internally? It isn't easy, since you can neither see nor estimate the amount of lost blood, as you can with an external hemorrhage. But one way you can tell is by detecting signs and symptoms of hypovolemic shock, as explained on pages 40 and 41.

For specific signs that'll help you determine the location of the bleeding, study the chart below. It'll also offer you *specific* care guidelines. Follow these general guidelines in *any* case of internal bleeding:

- Make sure the patient's airway remains open.
- Closely monitor his vital signs, including central venous pressure (CVP).
- Provide fluid replacement by administering any fluids (including blood) the doctor orders.
- Prepare the patient for surgery, if indicated. Remember to watch for hemorrhagic complications after surgery.
- Give the proper antidote if the patient's on anticoagulant therapy.

Important: Don't forget to support the patient and his family and explain what's happening.

Site	Specific signs and symptoms	Specific nursing care
Thorax	• Severe respiratory distress • Cardiac arrhythmias	• Elevate the head of the bed to ease your patient's breathing. • Administer oxygen, as needed. • Prepare to assist the doctor with chest tube insertion. After the procedure, check the color and amount of drainage every 15 minutes. Document it. Notify the doctor if the drainage shows frank (bright red) bleeding. If chest tube cannot be inserted immediately, the doctor may insert a flutter valve. • If the patient has a cardiac arrhythmia, make sure he's monitored. Treat arrhythmias as the doctor orders.
Abdomen	• Abdominal distention • Rigid, boardlike abdomen that's tender to the touch • Possible rebound abdominal tenderness • Vomiting, paralytic ileus, numbness and pain in legs, and lower back hematoma from retroperitoneal bleeding	• If hemorrhage is caused by a bleeding gastric ulcer, the doctor may order a gastric ice lavage to be administered via a nasogastric tube. • Be prepared to give cimetidine (Tagamet*), 300 mg diluted in 100 ml of I.V. solution given over 15 to 20 minutes every 6 hours, to decrease gastric bleeding. • Be prepared to assist the doctor with paracentesis.
Pelvis	• Abdominal or pelvic distention • Lower abdominal pain and tenderness • Lower back pain, in cases of renal involvement • Bloody urine • Decreased urine output	• If the patient's pelvis is fractured, prepare him for surgery or traction, as indicated. • Immobilize with a pelvic sling immediately to prevent further injury. • Insert Foley catheter, and observe urine output for amount and color. *Caution:* Never insert a Foley catheter if you suspect your patient's suffered urethral trauma. • If the patient's bleeding from the genitourinary tract, the doctor may want you to irrigate the patient's bladder with normal saline solution.
Thigh	• Erythema on affected leg • Painful, boardlike thigh that's tender to the touch • Localized edema and change in leg size	• Apply ice packs to affected area. • Elevate the affected leg. • Apply plastic air splint to affected area.

*Available in the United States and in Canada.

Hemorrhage

Understanding and dealing with hypovolemic shock

Anytime a patient loses a large amount of body fluid—as he would with a severe hemorrhage—he runs the risk of developing hypovolemic shock. To reverse this potentially lethal complication, if it occurs, you must give prompt, effective emergency care. Do you know how? Check your skills on the chart below.

Signs and symptoms
• Cold, clammy, or pale skin
• Low blood pressure
• Decreased temperature
• Increased pulse
• Increased respiration rate
• Blood and fluid loss exceeds 20% of total circulatory volume
• Restlessness
Physiologic changes
• Vasoconstriction, reducing blood flow to vital organs
• Inadequate oxygenation of individual cells (tissue perfusion)
• Increased lactic acid
• Impaired renal and hepatic function
• Metabolic acidosis

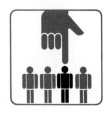

Caring for specific problems: Some tips

Sometimes a patient who's hemorrhaging severely has problems that require special attention. For example:

If he's on anticoagulant or aspirin therapy:
• Give the appropriate antidote, as prescribed by the doctor. To neutralize 75 to 90 units of heparin, give 1 mg protamine sulfate*, diluted 1%, I.V. push over 1 to 3 minutes. To neutralize warfarin sodium (Coumadin*), give 2.5 to 10 mg vitamin K_1* (phytonadione) I.M., subcutaneously, or I.V. push not to exceed 1 mg per minute.

If he's bleeding from a major abdominal vessel:
• Don't administer I.V. fluid in either leg. Why? Because the infusing I.V. fluid may escape from the damaged vessel into abdominal or retroperitoneal space.

If his neck is injured:
• Give I.V. fluids in the arm that's on the opposite side of the neck injury. Why? To keep the infusing I.V. fluid from leaving the damaged vessel and entering the intracranial or the thoracic space.

If he's hemorrhaging from a fractured arm or leg:
• Apply a plastic air splint to provide pressure and to immobilize the fracture. (For details, see page 37.)

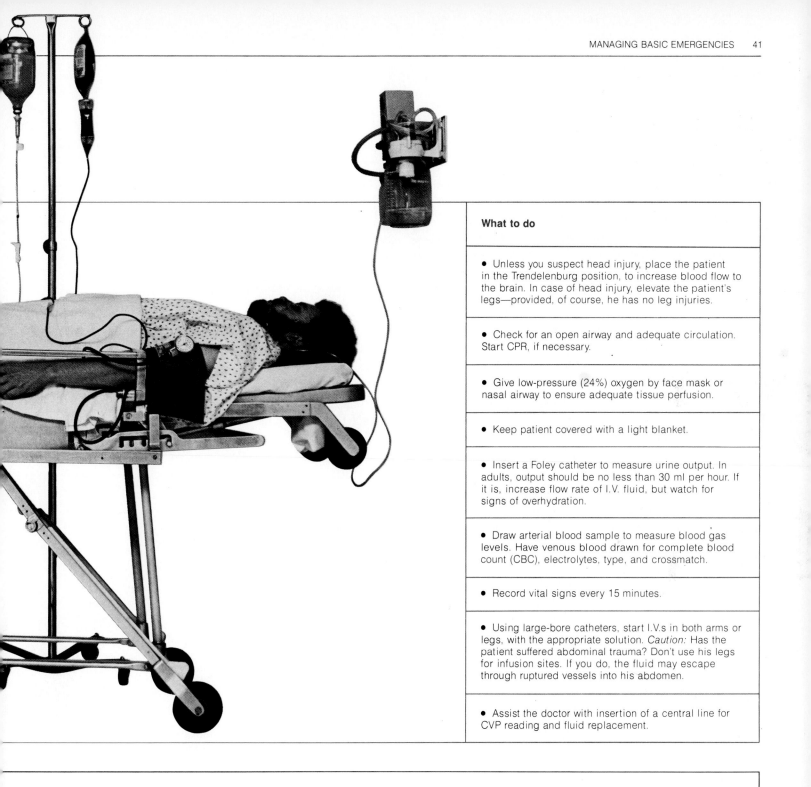

What to do

- Unless you suspect head injury, place the patient in the Trendelenburg position, to increase blood flow to the brain. In case of head injury, elevate the patient's legs—provided, of course, he has no leg injuries.

- Check for an open airway and adequate circulation. Start CPR, if necessary.

- Give low-pressure (24%) oxygen by face mask or nasal airway to ensure adequate tissue perfusion.

- Keep patient covered with a light blanket.

- Insert a Foley catheter to measure urine output. In adults, output should be no less than 30 ml per hour. If it is, increase flow rate of I.V. fluid, but watch for signs of overhydration.

- Draw arterial blood sample to measure blood gas levels. Have venous blood drawn for complete blood count (CBC), electrolytes, type, and crossmatch.

- Record vital signs every 15 minutes.

- Using large-bore catheters, start I.V.s in both arms or legs, with the appropriate solution. *Caution:* Has the patient suffered abdominal trauma? Don't use his legs for infusion sites. If you do, the fluid may escape through ruptured vessels into his abdomen.

- Assist the doctor with insertion of a central line for CVP reading and fluid replacement.

- Avoid raising the fractured limb, as this may damage the bone, the vessel, or the surrounding tissue.

If he has hemophilia:
- Depending on the doctor's orders, administer one or all of the following: plasma, vitamin K₁, or antihemophilic factor (AHF), 10 to 20 units/kg, I.V. push or infusion every 8 to 24 hours.
- Never give aspirin, or any drug containing aspirin, for pain.
- Use a finger stick to draw blood for coagulation studies.
- If your patient refuses needed blood or blood products because of personal or religious beliefs, consider giving a plasma expander, like dextran I.V., per doctor's order. If the patient's a minor, the doctor may request a court order for permission to perform the appropriate lifesaving treatment.

If your patient develops disseminated intravascular coagulation (DIC):
- Observe him closely for occult bleeding.
- Give plasma, platelets, or packed red blood cells, per doctor's order.
- If a blood transfusion proves ineffective, give anticoagulant therapy I.V., per doctor's order. However, before giving an anticoagulant, check the patient's blood coagulation studies for baseline information. Expect the prothrombin time (PT) and the partial thromboplastin time (PTT) to be prolonged in the late stages of DIC.

*Available in the United States and in Canada.

Hemorrhage

How to remove a MAST suit

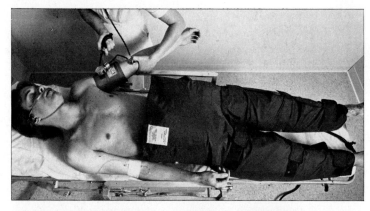

1 *You're working in the ED when car accident victim Frank Berry is brought in wearing Medical Anti-shock Trousers (a MAST suit). From the emergency medical technician you find out that Frank has a severed artery in his left leg. Because of this, he's lost massive amounts of blood, and has only a palpable blood pressure, both signs of hypovolemic shock. What do you do next? Do you know how to remove a MAST suit? If you're not sure, read this photostory.*

First, take Frank's blood pressure to get a baseline reading for later use. Then, check his apical heart rate.

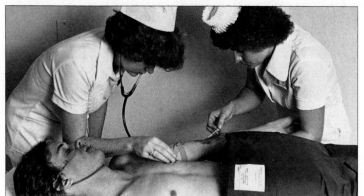

2 While you're taking Frank's vital signs, have another nurse insert two large-bore catheters (16G or larger) into his arms to begin fluid replacement. At the same time, draw blood for type and crossmatch. Check the skin color and temperature of Frank's feet, and feel for pedal pulses. (Remember, you can expect pedal pulses to be faint when the MAST suit is properly inflated.)

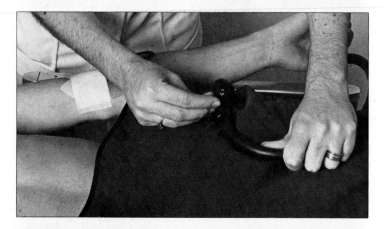

3 When Frank's condition has stabilized, the doctor may decide you can remove the MAST suit. Here's how. First, take a close look at the suit's construction. Does it have separate chambers for the legs and abdomen? If it does, open the stopcock on the abdominal compartment, as the nurse is doing here, and release a small amount of pressure.

Immediately check Frank's blood pressure. If it's dropped 30 or more points from your baseline reading, the doctor may order a fluid challenge. Perform this by increasing the I.V. flow rate 100 to 200 ml over the next 10 minutes. In most cases, the increased flow rate will bring your patient's blood pressure back to an acceptable level. Then, you can continue deflating the abdominal compartment of the MAST suit gradually, with regular blood pressure checks—and any necessary fluid challenges—after each deflation.

Suppose the fluid challenge doesn't bring Frank's blood pressure up. Alert the doctor immediately, as you reinflate the MAST suit.

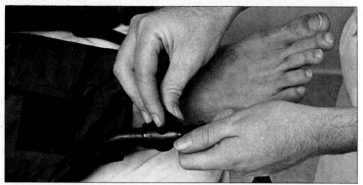

4 When you've completely deflated the abdominal compartment of Frank's MAST suit, wait approximately 5 minutes so his body can adjust to the loss of external pressure. Then, begin deflating the leg compartments of the suit, leaving the *left* compartment—the leg with the severed artery—till last. Check Frank's blood pressure after each deflation, and perform any necessary fluid challenges (see earlier instructions). At this point, the doctor can repair the severed artery.

Important: Conflicting medical opinions exist concerning which leg compartment to deflate first, or whether to deflate both simultaneously. Always check and follow *your* hospital's policy before attempting to remove a MAST suit.

AT THE SCENE

How to apply a tourniquet

1 *Picture yourself at the scene of an accident. You see that the victim has arterial bleeding from a leg amputation. Your quick assessment—following the guidelines on page 8—assures you that she doesn't need artificial respiration. So you try applying direct and indirect pressure to her wound to control the bleeding. When nothing works, you realize you'll have to use a tourniquet. This photostory will show you how.*

Caution: Since you risk the loss of your patient's limb when you use a tourniquet, apply one only in an extreme emergency; for example, if she's injured a large artery.

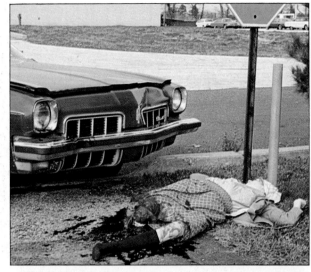

2 First, locate the artery that controls blood flow to the injury. In this case, it's the femoral artery. Then, place a pad of folded material—whatever's handy—directly over the site, between the patient's heart and the wound.

Next, use a stocking, scarf, belt, or large handkerchief to make a tourniquet. Wrap it around the patient's thigh, covering the pad, and tie the ends in a half-knot, as shown here. Never use wire or cord, which could cause tissue damage.

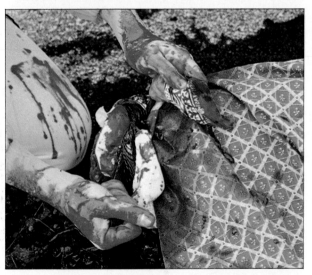

3 Now, take a stick or similar item, and center it over the half-knot. Tie a square knot over the stick, and tighten the tourniquet by twisting the stick.

Does the bleeding increase? You may be applying only enough pressure to obstruct venous return not arterial flow. Make the tourniquet tighter.

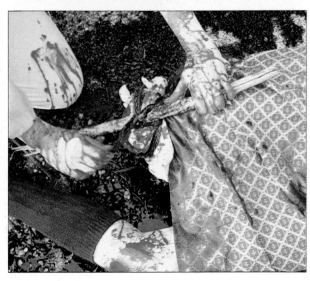

4 Once the tourniquet's in place, apply a sterile dressing or clean cloth directly over the wound. Be careful not to disturb any blood clots. If possible, elevate the affected leg or arm. Get the patient to a hospital immediately.

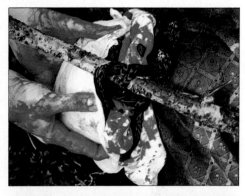

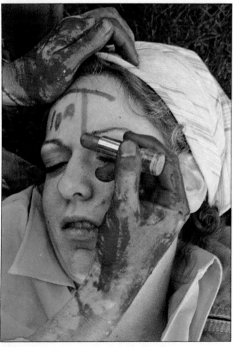

5 *Important:* Make sure the ambulance personnel and the hospital staff know the patient has a tourniquet. Use a lipstick or pen to make a large *T* on her forehead, as shown here. Or fasten a tag on her stating the location of the tourniquet and the time of application.

Be sure the severed limb accompanies the patient to the hospital. *Remember:* Replantation may be possible. Place the limb in a plastic bag and, if available, cover with ice. Don't let the limb come directly in contact with the ice. For more details on how to care for a traumatic amputation, see pages 102 and 103.

Burn care

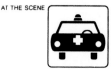

Chances are, you'll probably have to give emergency care to a patient with burn injuries someday. When that time comes, will you be ready to give the skilled nursing care he needs? Do you know, for example, how to assess a burn injury's severity? What's your first priority in dealing with chemical, electrical, or thermal burns? How about decontaminating a patient with radiation burns? The answers to these and many other questions nurses commonly ask about burns can be found on the following pages.

How to care for thermal burns

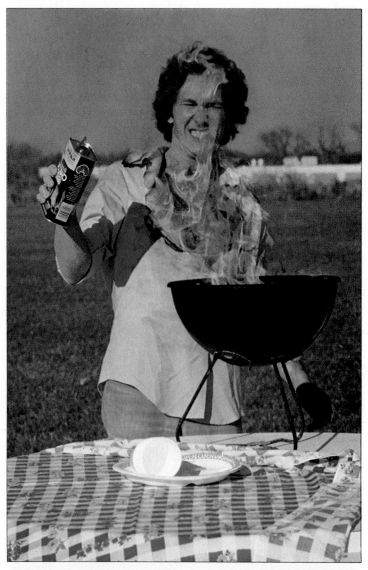

1 *You're attending an outdoor barbecue when your neighbor, Chuck Sands, pours lighter fluid on red-hot charcoal briquettes. Instantly, flames flash from the grill and ignite Mr. Sands' clothes. What do you do?*

Act quickly. First, make him lie down. Don't let him run in panic, as this will fan the flames, prolong his contact with heat, and increase the risk of inhalation injury.

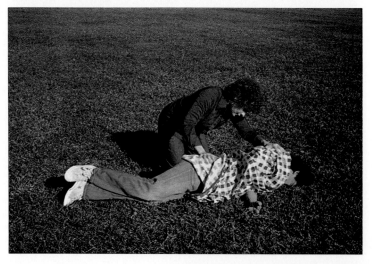

2 Smother the flames by logrolling Mr. Sands in a tablecloth, coat, or whatever's available. *Important:* Don't use sand or dirt to extinguish flames; you may contaminate the burn injuries.

3 If water's nearby, use it to douse the flames, as shown here. Water will also help cool the burn quickly.

Remove any jewelry Mr. Sands is wearing on the burned area, to prevent further tissue damage from hot metal. This will also prevent impaired circulation from edema. Also, remove any smoldering clothing if you can't cool them with water. *Caution:* Never apply ice to a burn, because the extreme cold could cause additional tissue damage.

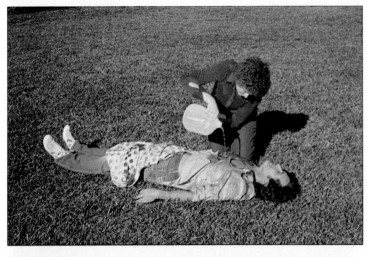

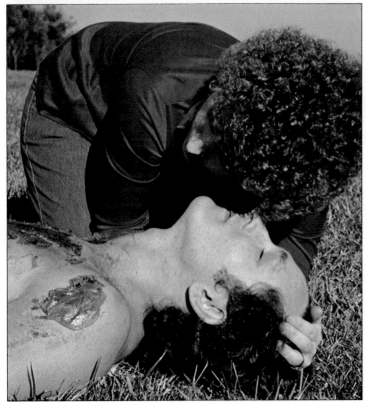

4 Now, do an emergency assessment (ABCs) to check Mr. Sands' airway, breathing, and circulation. Also check him for other injuries; for example, fractures, lacerations, or chest wounds. Make sure someone's called for an ambulance.

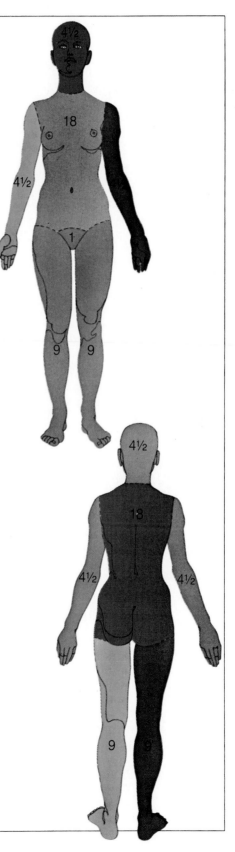

5 In the meantime, assess the burn's severity by using the Rule of Nines. As you know, this method divides body surface area (BSA) into areas representing 9 or multiples of 9%, as shown in this diagram. To use this technique at the scene, quickly examine the burns, as you mentally picture the diagram. Imagine shading the areas where your patient's burned. Then, total these percentages to get a rough estimate of the burn involvement. *Remember:* Be sure to give this information to the emergency medical technicians when they arrive. It'll help them determine what specific lifesaving measures to take as they transport the patient to the hospital.

Burn care

How to care for thermal burns continued

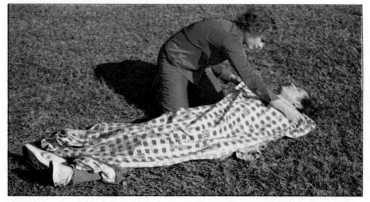

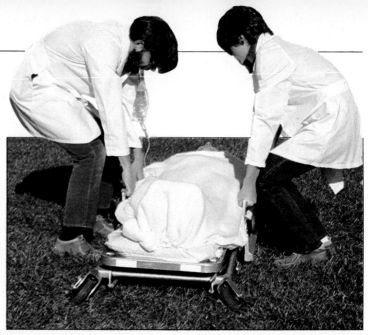

6 When the patient's been burned severely, metabolic changes and loss of his skin's protective function can cause his body temperature to drop dramatically. So, cover him with a clean sheet or towel, or whatever's available. This will help guard against wound contamination and pain caused by air currents.

7 Stay with Mr. Sands until the ambulance arrives to transport him to the ED. Continue checking his airway, breathing, and circulation. Reassure the patient as much as possible. Don't permit anyone to give him anything to drink.

How severe is your patient's burn injury?

MINI-ASSESSMENT

As you know, to determine a burn injury's severity, you have to assess its size and depth. To do this, ask yourself these questions:

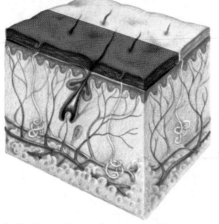

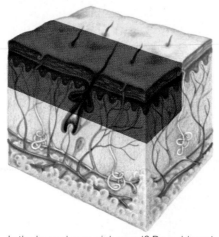

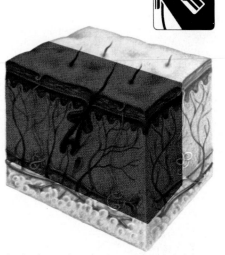

Is the burned area pink or red, with minimal edema? Is it painful to touch and sensitive to temperature change? If so, your patient has a first-degree burn, involving one or two layers of skin (partial thickness).

Is the burned area pink or red? Do reddened areas blanch when touched? Does the patient have large, thick-walled blisters, with considerable subcutaneous edema? Is the burned area firm or leathery? When you touch the burn, does the patient have severe pain? If so, he has a second-degree burn, involving at least two layers of skin (partial thickness).

Is the burned area waxy white, red, brown, or black? If red, does the burn remain red, with no blanching, when touched? Is it leathery, with extensive subcutaneous edema? Insensitive to touch? If so, your patient has a third-degree burn, involving all skin layers (full thickness).

Remember: Consider *any* second- or third-degree burn serious in the following cases:
• your patient is over age 60 or under 2.
• your patient has a disease that compromises his ability to manage fluid shifts and to resist infection (for example, diabetes mellitus, congestive heart failure, cirrhosis), or has renal, respiratory, or gastrointestinal problems.
• your patient's hands, feet, or genitals are involved.
• your patient's burn covers 10% or more of his total body surface area; 5% or more if he's a child.

In the ED: Caring for the patient with thermal burns

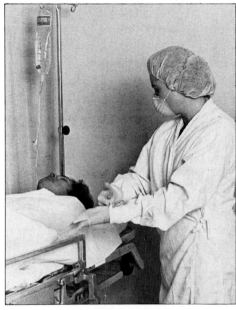

1 *Let's assume you're working in the ED when 28-year-old Chuck Sands arrives with second- and third-degree burns over 15% of his body. He's received emergency care at the scene and has an I.V. in place. Do you know what to do next? Follow these steps:*

First, don a sterile gown, cap, mask, and gloves, as shown here. Reassure your patient that you're going to help him, and explain each procedure.

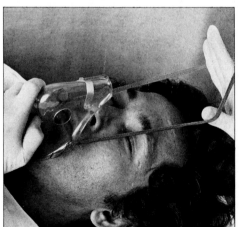

2 Make sure he has an open airway. Administer humidified oxygen, if needed, and have a trach tray handy, in case of emergency. If severe respiratory distress occurs, or you see signs of inhalation injury (singed nasal hairs or black sputum), he will have to be intubated. (For full details on how to do this, see the NURSING PHOTOBOOK *Providing Respiratory Care.)*

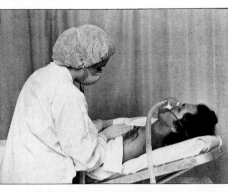

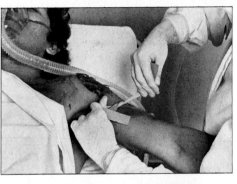

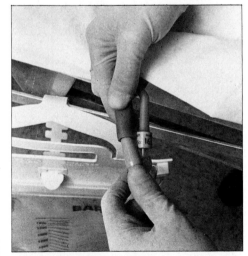

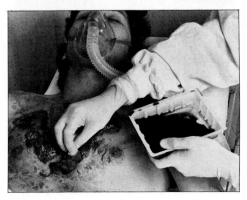

3 Now, check your patient's blood pressure, apical heart rate, peripheral pulses, respirations, and temperature. If his blood pressure is normal, elevate his head and upper torso, as shown here.

4 Using the Berkow method, explained on page 49, quickly assess the extent of your patient's burns, and record your findings. Then, insert a second large-bore catheter for I.V. therapy, as ordered. At the same time, draw a blood sample for the necessary diagnostic tests, which include complete blood count (CBC), type and crossmatch, creatinine, blood urea nitrogen (BUN), total serum protein, albumin, globulin, and electrolytes. Also draw an arterial blood sample for blood gas measurements.

5 The doctor will want you to insert a Foley catheter. (For details on how to insert a Foley catheter, see page 86.) When you do, be sure to get a urine sample for urinalysis. Then, when the patient's condition has stabilized, make sure he has a chest X-ray and an electrocardiogram. Obtain and document all the information you need about your patient, as well as the accident, so it can accompany him when he's transferred to another unit. For instructions on what to include, see page 48.

6 Before your patient leaves the ED, use sterile gauze and a mild antiseptic solution to remove any gross debris from his burns. Remember, he'll get a more thorough wound cleansing later, in the burn unit.

Administer tetanus toxoid prophylactically, after checking first to make sure he's not allergic to it.

To prevent wound contamination and possible pain caused by circulating air, cover your patient with a sterile sheet or blanket. *Nursing tip:* Use a space blanket, readily available from sporting good stores, to keep your patient warm during transfer.

Burn care

Documenting emergency burn care properly

To document the care you give a burn patient in the ED, you must collect as much information as you can about the accident, the patient's past medical history, and his present physical condition. Use a data collection sheet like the one shown here, and fill in every blank.

Find out how the burn occurred and what kind of care was given to the patient before he arrived at the hospital. Ask if he's been taking any medication or has any chronic illnesses, or allergies. Record the baseline data you'll get from various diagnostic tests.

Take time to record specific information accurately. The healthcare professionals who care for him later will need all the information you can provide. Then, make sure the properly filled out data collection sheet accompanies him when he's transferred.

AGE: _28_
SEX: _Male_
TIME OF BURN: _1:30 PM_

NAME: _Chuck Sands_
HOSPITAL NO.: _78910_
ADMISSION DATE: _9/24/79 2 PM_

BURN ASSESSMENT SHEET

	INTAKE	DATE TIME	2 PM	3 PM	4 PM		MEDICATION	TIME
		Temperature	96	97	97⁴		P.O./I.M.	
		Pulse	112	110	116		9/24 0.5 Tetanus Toxoid	2:30 P.M. D.J.
		Resp.	24	22	22			
		B.P.	100/80	110/60	112/64			
		O₂ therapy	85% 100%	40%	40%			
		CVP	—	6	6⁵			
		Hematocrit	—	—	—			
		Oral	—	—	—			
		Dextrose	—	60	120			
		Saline	—	—	—			
		Hartmann's with 25 gm salt poor albumin	900	900	750		9/24	
		Blood	—	—	—		I.V. 5 mill. units Penicillin IV	3:00 PM H.N.
		Plasma	—	—	—		10 mg. Morphine Sulphate IV	3:30 PM H.N.
		Medication in dextrose	—	100	—			
		TOTAL	900	1060	870			
		SHIFT TOTAL	900	—	1930			
	OUTPUT	Urine	—	100	95			
		GI	120	20	30			
		Other/stool	—	—	—			
		TOTAL	120	120	125			
		SHIFT TOTAL	120	—	245			
		Specific Gravity	1.024	—	1.018			
		Sugar/Acetone	N/TR		N/+1			
		Protein/pH	+2/6⁵		+2/6			

NURSES' NOTES 2 PM - 28-year-old male admitted with thermal burns of approximately 15% of body. Burn sustained after pouring lighter fluid on hot charcoal in grill. Patient conscious and extremely apprehensive. 2:15 PM Baseline arterial blood gas sample obtained and sent to lab. Dr. Jones intubated pt. with #8 oral E.T. O₂ started @ 40% with high humidity. 2:25 PM #18 Salem Sump tube inserted - 120 ml. dark green fluid hematest ⊕ obtained. SS attached to low intermittent suction. 2:30 PM - I.V. catheter inserted in R subclavian. 1000 ml Hartmann's c 25 gm Salt Poor Albumin added at 15 ml/min via infusion pump. Blood obtained for baseline CBC, electrolytes, PT, PTT. 2:40 PM #18g IV catheter inserted in left antecubital space. — 1000 ML. D₅W at 15 gtts/min. 2:45 PM - #16 Foley catheter inserted and attached to Urine-meter. Specimen sent to lab. Sample hematest ⊕
— Dorothy Jovinelly R.N.

3 PM Hair shaved around burned areas on chest and arms. 3:20 Pt. appears restless, more agitated and c/o severe pain. Repeat ABG's obtained. D₅/W rate increased to 30 gtts/min. as ordered. 3:30 Morphine Sulphate 10mg IV given. Helene Nawrocki R N
3:35 Burned areas cleansed with Betadine scrub. Pt. prepared for transfer to Burn Treatment Center. 4 PM Transferred via stretcher to 4th Floor BTC, accompanied by R N
— Helene Nawrocki R N

Using the Berkow method to document burn injuries

Before transferring your patient to a burn unit, make sure you document the extent of his burn injury. You can do this with the Berkow method, illustrated here. Here's how:

• First, shade the body diagrams to match the burned areas on your patient's body.

• Next, record the numbers appearing in those shaded areas in the appropriate columns to the right. Is only a fraction of an area burned? Divide that fraction into the number, and record the answer.

• Remember, as a child grows, his body proportions change. Most notably, such changes occur in his head, thighs, and legs. The percentage of the body that these areas represent varies according to age. To calculate it correctly, use the chart at the bottom of the illustration.

• Now, add all the numbers you've recorded, to arrive at the subtotals. Then, add these subtotals to determine the final total, which is the approximate percentage of body surface area burned. *Important:* Don't forget to gauge the depth as well as the size of the burn when assessing its severity. (To gauge depth correctly, see page 46.)

AGE: _28_
SEX: _Male_
WEIGHT: _135 lbs._
HEIGHT: _5'7"_

NAME: _Chuck Sauds_
HOSPITAL: _Centerville Hospital_
DATE: _9/24/79 2 P.M._
FORM COMPLETED BY: _Dorothy Gourmally RN_

ESTIMATION OF SIZE OF BURN BY PERCENT

1. COLOR IN THE BURN

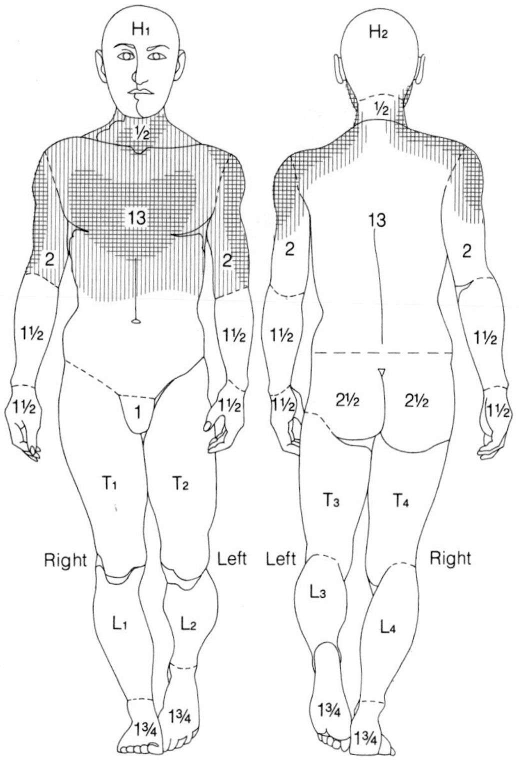

ANTERIOR — POSTERIOR

Partial thickness | Full thickness

CALCULATE EXTENT BURN

	ANTERIOR	POSTERIOR
Head	H_1 0	H_2 0
Neck	½	¼
Rt. Arm	2	½
Rt. Forearm	0	0
Rt. Hand	0	0
Lt. Arm	2	½
Lt. Forearm	0	0
Lt. Hand	0	0
Trunk	9	¼
Buttock	(R) 0	(L) 0
Perineum	0	0
Rt. Thigh	T_1 0	T_4 0
Rt. Leg	L_1 0	L_4 0
Rt. Foot	0	0
Lt. Thigh	T_2 0	T_3 0
Lt. Leg	L_2 0	L_3 0
Lt. Foot	0	0
Subtotal	13½	1½

% Total area burned _15_

2. CIRCLE AGE FACTOR		Percent of areas affected by growth					
AGE		0	1	5	10	15	Adult
H(1 or 2)= ½ of the Head		9½	8½	6½	5½	4½	3½
T(1, 2, 3, or 4)= ½ of a Thigh		2¾	3¼	4	4¼	4¼	4¾
L(1, 2, 3, or 4)= ½ of a Leg		2½	2½	2¾	3	3¼	3½

Burn care

How burn injuries can cause hypovolemic shock

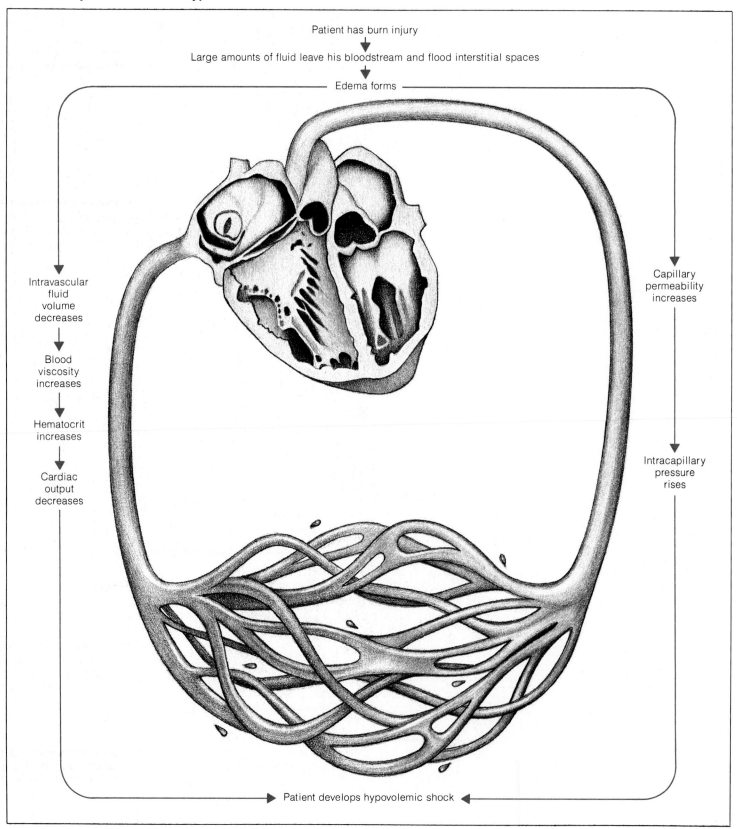

Patient has burn injury

Large amounts of fluid leave his bloodstream and flood interstitial spaces

Edema forms

Intravascular
fluid
volume
decreases

Blood
viscosity
increases

Hematocrit
increases

Cardiac
output
decreases

Capillary
permeability
increases

Intracapillary
pressure
rises

Patient develops hypovolemic shock

Dealing with frostbite

Frostbite is another type of thermal burn you'll care for occasionally, especially if you work in an area where winters are severe. In most cases, you can recognize frostbite on a patient's arms, legs, or face by checking for the following: white or mottled blue-white skin that's hard to the touch, blisters, and complaints of numbness in affected area.

To care for the patient properly, first immerse the frostbitten arm or leg in warm water (99° to 103° F. [37.2° to 39° C.]). If the affected area is on his face, apply moist, warm towels. Wait several minutes for the frozen area to thaw. As it does, the patient will regain sensation in that area and probably complain of severe pain. In addition, the affected area will look flushed and feel warm.

Discontinue the warm water immersion or towel applications. Administer tetanus toxoid and whatever sedatives or analgesics the doctor's ordered, checking first to make sure the patient's not allergic to them.

Look for other injuries, and find out if your patient has any chronic illnesses that may affect subsequent treatment.

Document the size and color of the affected area in your nurses' notes, as well as your care, information about his medical history, and the circumstances surrounding the injury.

Warn your patient and his family that he must be especially careful not to let the affected area get too cold in the future. Permanent tissue damage can result if previously frostbitten areas become frozen again.

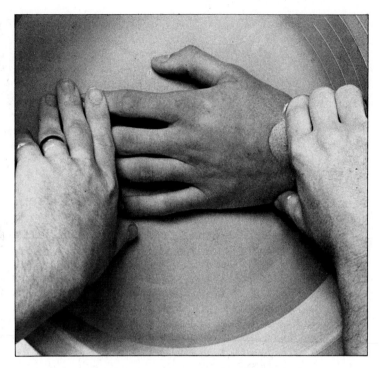

AT THE SCENE

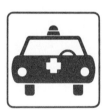

How to care for chemical burns

In most cases, chemical burns result from home or industrial accidents. Tissue damage is usually caused by direct chemical action and its subsequent release of heat energy. The burn's severity depends on the chemical's concentration and the length of time it remains on the victim's skin. No wonder, then, that your prompt, effective action is so important if you're at the scene of the accident. Here's what to do:

First, immediately dilute the chemical by flushing the burned area with copious amounts of water or normal saline solution, as shown here. Then, remove any clothing surrounding the burned area. This will prevent further tissue damage from chemicals that remain in your patient's garments.

Find out which chemical or combination of chemicals caused his burn. Make sure this information is documented so other health-care professionals can begin specific treatment when your patient arrives in the emergency department. Check the patient for any other injuries and document these also. Continue flushing the burn until you transport him to the ED, or he's no longer in your care.

Important: Never flush a phosphorus burn with water or any type of solution. Doing so could cause tissue sloughing. Instead, gently soak the affected area with water.

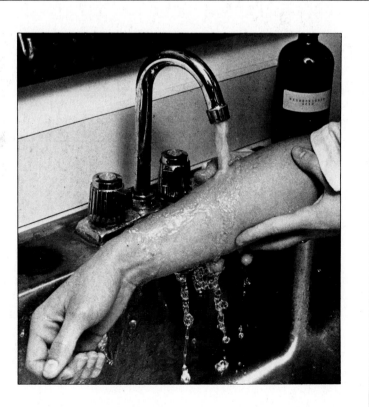

Burn care

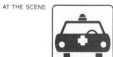

How to care for electrical burns

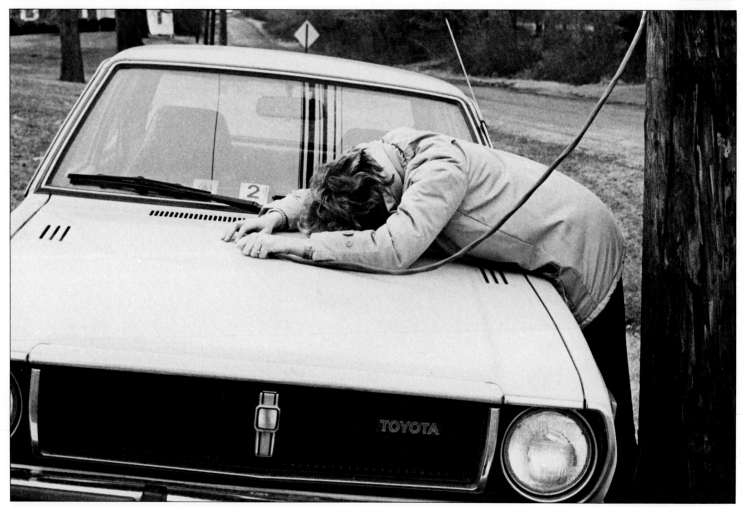

1 Imagine this situation: You and a co-worker are on your way home after a busy night. Along the side of the road, you see a young woman about to remove a high-voltage wire that's fallen on her car. Before you can warn her, she grabs the wire. Do you know what to do? If not, review these steps:

First, you and your co-worker should stay clear of the victim, the car, and the wire. *Caution:* Never touch anyone who's receiving an electrical shock. Doing so may endanger your own life.

As you keep bystanders away from the accident, have your co-worker notify the power company and the rescue squad.

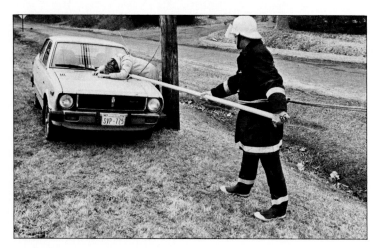

2 Suppose the rescue department arrives before the power company. Because the victim is showing signs of cardiac arrest, they decide to separate the victim from the wire before the power is shut off. Here's how they'll proceed:

First, rescue personnel will tie a rope around the rescuer's waist. That way the rescuer can be removed from the power source in case of unexpected difficulties. When the rope's secured, the rescuer will put on rubber insulated boots and gloves.

Then, using an 8' (240 cm) fiberglass pole, the rescuer will push the wire away from the victim, as shown here.

How to care for radiation burns

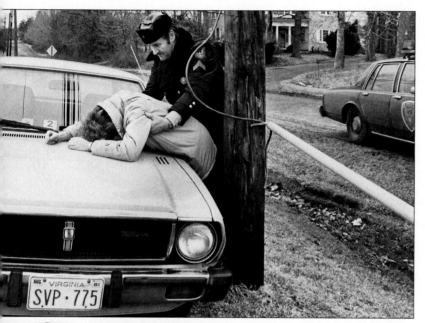

3 As the first rescuer uses the pole to hold the wire clear of the victim and car, a second rescuer gently removes the victim from the car.

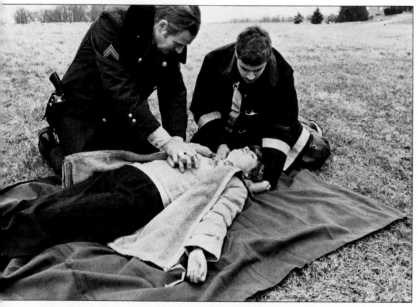

4 When the victim's successfully separated from the electrical current, rescue personnel do a quick emergency assessment (ABCs) and check her vital signs. Give artificial respiration and cardiopulmonary resuscitation (CPR), if needed. Always ensure an open airway, and treat possible cardiac arrest *before* you care for the victim's electrical burns. Then, as soon as possible get her to the ED.

There, the entrance and exit wounds will be treated as thermal burns. Keep in mind that electrical burns never look as bad as they are. For example, the victim may have only minimal *external* tissue damage, but considerable *internal* damage along nerve and vascular pathways.

Caring for a radiation burn victim? You'll have to make special provisions before and after he arrives. Why? Because radioactive contamination, usually present in such a burn, creates a serious health hazard for all who come in contact with the victim. *Remember:* Radioactive decontamination guidelines differ, so always follow your state's and hospital's policies. Also keep in mind that this information *does not apply* to patient's suffering skin irritation from radiation therapy.

Here's how to prepare for the victim's arrival:
• Prepare an isolated area in which to treat him. Make sure there's enough room for health-care professionals, disposal hampers, and the stretcher. Enclose the area with lead-lined shields. If that's impossible, make arrangements to care for the patient in your hospital's X-ray department. Next, cover the floor of the area with newspapers or other absorbent paper. Tape the paper in place with masking tape.
• Notify hospital maintenance personnel that you may want to shut off the air-circulating system in the area.
• Make sure you and the other team members are wearing surgical caps, masks, gowns, gloves, and booties.

After the victim arrives, follow these steps:
• Use a Geiger counter to check his contamination level while he's still on the ambulance stretcher. Then, get him to the shielded area immediately.
• When he's inside the area, do a quick head-to-toe assessment, using the guidelines explained in Section 1. Treat any life-threatening injuries and administer tetanus toxoid, as ordered.
• Save any clothes you remove from the patient, as well as the bedding from the ambulance. Also, save any metal objects the patient is wearing, such as jewelry, a belt buckle, or dental appliances. Instruct another health-care professional to label each item with the patient's name, his location within the hospital, the date, and the time. Retain each item in an individual lead or plastic container that's been clearly marked RADIOACTIVE: DO NOT DISCARD.
• If you suspect the patient may have inhaled or ingested radioactive materials, save any blood, urine, or vomitus. Place it in an individual container and label as explained above.
• Cleanse radiation burns with soap and water. If the patient's entire body is contaminated, shower him in a lead-lined shower. When you cleanse your patient, pay special attention to hairy body surfaces, orifices, and skin folds.
• To decontaminate your patient, you'll probably have to wash or shower him several times. Measure and record his contamination level each time. Continue until the contamination level registers zero on the Geiger counter.
• Transfer the radiation burn patient to the proper unit, where his burns will be treated like thermal burns. After that, you'll have to decontaminate yourself and anyone else who's been in contact with him. To do this, follow the steps above.

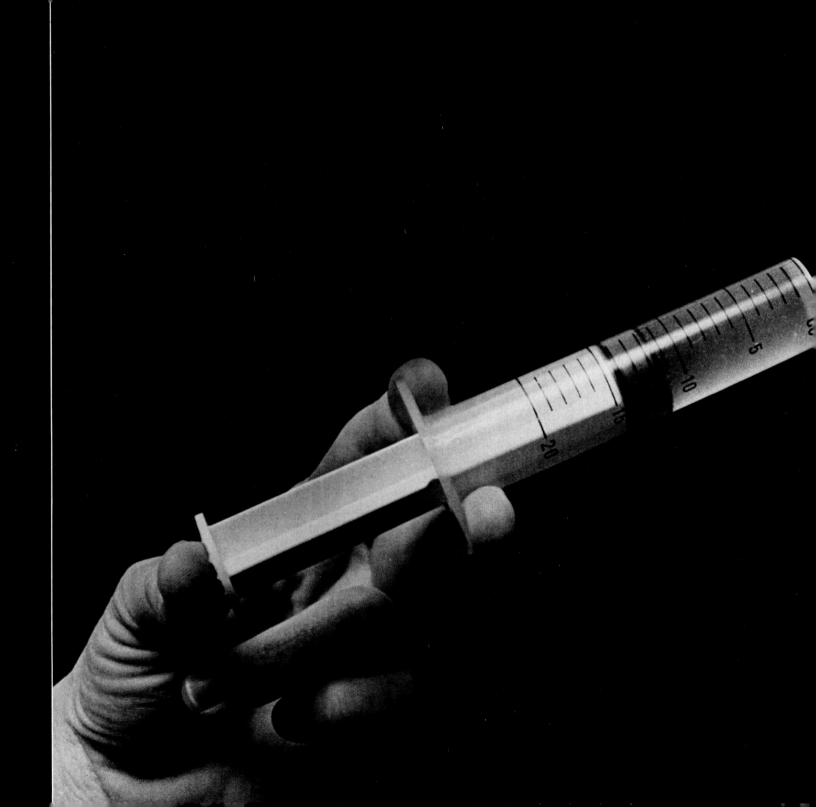

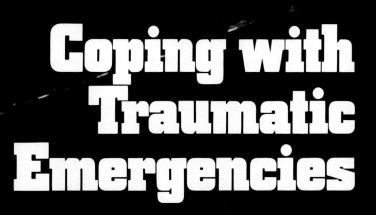

Coping with Traumatic Emergencies

EENT emergencies

Cardiopulmonary emergencies

Abdominal/pelvic emergencies

Arm and leg emergencies

EENT emergencies

Caring for a patient with a traumatic injury to the eyes, ears, nose, or throat? You'll have to assess his injury quickly.

Does your patient have an eye infection? He may need an eye irrigation to help treat it. Is he wearing contact lenses? You may have to remove them. And, if the doctor orders an eye patch, you must know how to apply one properly.

What if your patient has a foreign body in his ear? Do you know how and when to do an irrigation?

Suppose your patient has a severe nosebleed that can't be controlled by the usual methods. Can you help the doctor insert an anterior/posterior nasal pack, if needed? Do you know how to assist the doctor?

On these pages you'll find step-by-step instructions for all these procedures. Also, some nursing tips you'll want to remember.

How to inspect your patient's eyes

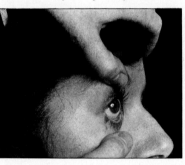

1 *When you inspect your patient's eyes, always check for contact lenses, foreign bodies, edema, drainage, ptosis, inflammations, corneal lacerations, or fractures of the bony orbit. (Obviously, you'll also want to check the patient's pupillary activity. To find out how, see page 132.)*

For the conditions listed above, proceed as follows. First, reassure your patient, and explain what you're going to do. Then, have her sit facing you in a well-lighted area.

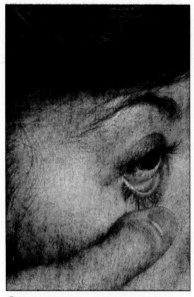

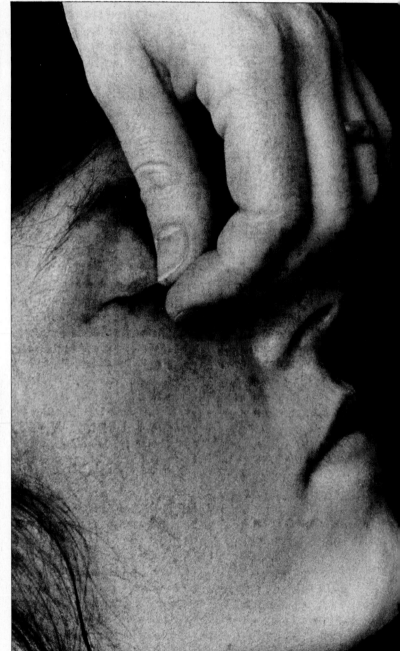

2 Start by palpating the bony orbits around both eyes. Document any suspected fractures.

Now, examine the conjunctiva and the eyeball of each eye, as follows. First, evert the lower lid by gently pulling it down over the lower orbital rim. Take care not to exert pressure on the eyeball. Then, ask your patient to look up, down, left, and right, in that order. Examine the area thoroughly.

3 To evert the upper lid, ask your patient to look down. Slightly raise her eyelid to make her eyelashes protrude. Now, with one hand, grasp the lashes and gently pull them down and forward.

4 With your other hand, place a cotton swab on top of the eyelid, just above the fold.

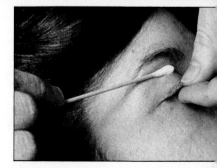

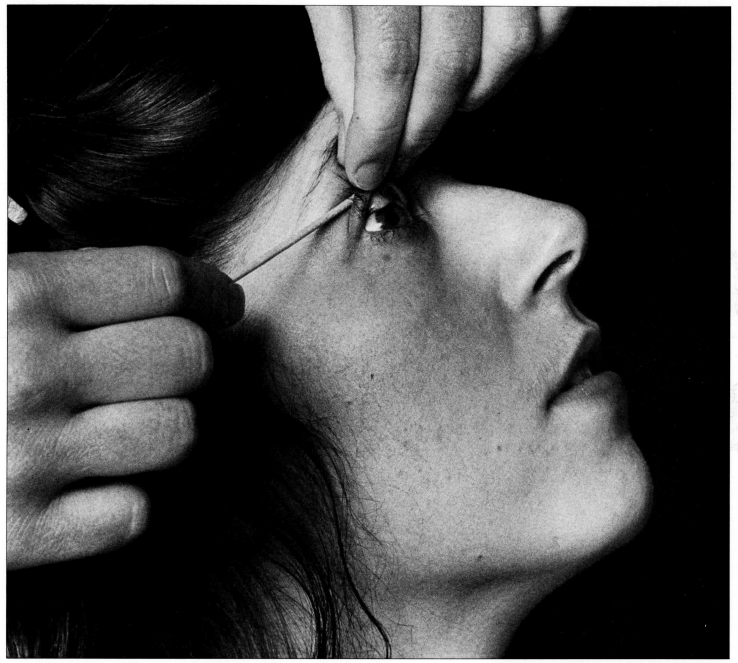

5 Roll the eyelid up over the cotton swab, as shown here. With one finger, secure the patient's eyelashes against the upper orbital rim. Examine the area thoroughly.

Return the eyelid to its normal position by asking the patient to look up while you gently pull forward on her eyelashes.

Repeat the entire procedure for the other eye, and document your findings. Except for small foreign bodies, which you can remove yourself, report any abnormalities to the doctor.

EENT emergencies

How to remove contact lenses

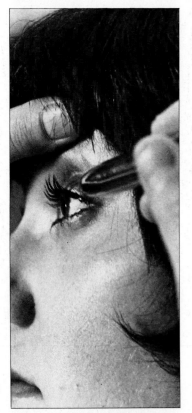

1 *Preparing to do an emergency eye examination? Make sure you ask your patient whether or not she's wearing contact lenses. If she is, have her remove them. Suppose she's unable to communicate with you for some reason. Check her eyes yourself, using a small flashlight.*

Gently open the patient's eyes, and shine a beam of light from the side, as shown here. If she's wearing hard contact lenses, you'll see an outline slightly smaller than her iris. With soft lenses, you'll see an outline covering the entire iris and sclera.

Now, remove any lenses that are present, using one of the following methods.

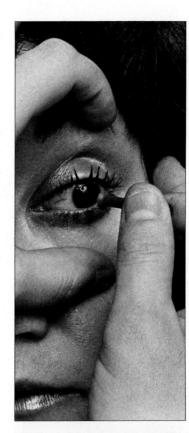

3 Suppose you're unable to remove a hard contact lens by popping it out. Use a small suction bulb especially designed for lens removal. But work carefully; don't let the suction bulb come in contact with the cornea, as it may cause permanent damage.

Gently place the cup end against the contact lens.

[Inset below] The lens will adhere to it as you pull the bulb away from the patient's eyeball in a straight line. Immediately place the lens in a properly labeled container, and repeat the procedure with the other eye.

Nursing tip: If no special suction bulb's available, use the tip of a glass eyedropper instead.

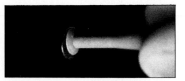

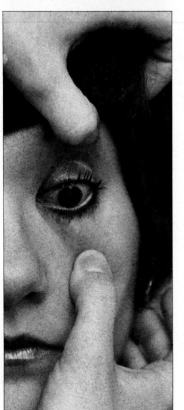

2 The first method we'll show is for hard lens removal. Start with the right eye and work gently. Standing to your patient's right, place your left thumb on her upper eyelid, and your right thumb on her lower eyelid. Pull the eyelids apart, wide enough to expose the contact lens completely.

Now, press down with your right thumb, tipping the lens forward. *Gently* pinch the patient's eyelids together to expel the lens. Carefully remove it, and place it in a container labeled with the patient's name and hospital identification number. Mark the container with an *R* to indicate the *right* lens. Repeat the procedure with the left eye, and mark the container with an *L*.

Important: Never use force when removing a contact lens. If you have difficulty, slide the lens onto the sclera, and call the doctor.

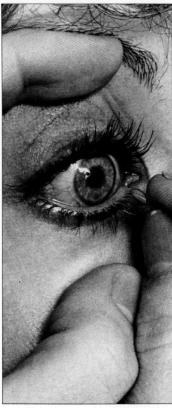

4 To remove a soft contact lens, place your index finger directly on the lens, and gently slide it down, away from the cornea. Lightly pinch the lens between your thumb and index finger, and lift it out. Completely immerse the lens in a properly labeled container of sterile *normal saline solution*, and repeat the procedure with the other eye. *Important:* Never use anything but normal saline solution to immerse soft lenses. Any other solution may permanently damage them.

Here's another way to remove a soft lens. With your index finger, gently retract the patient's lower eyelid until you can see the edge of the contact lens. Maintaining gentle pressure, stretch the skin slightly in the direction of the patient's ear. When her eyelid is directly under the contact lens, grasp the lens between your thumb and index finger and remove it.

How to irrigate your patient's eyes

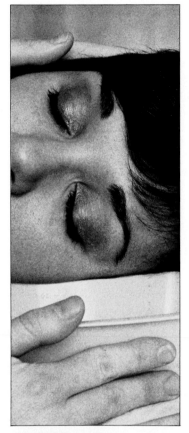

1 *You may need to irrigate your patient's eyes for any of these reasons: to prepare her for eye surgery, to treat infection, to remove secretions, or to flush away small foreign bodies or contaminants. Which irrigating solution the doctor orders depends, of course, on the patient's specific condition. Remember, before irrigating, instill a local anesthetic in your patient's eye, as ordered by the doctor.*

To perform the irrigation, first gather the necessary equipment: a plastic irrigation bottle or bulb syringe containing the prescribed solution, an emesis basin for drainage, an absorbent bedsaver pad, and a supply of gauze pads or cotton. Make sure the irrigating solution is room temperature.

Now, reassure your patient, and explain what you're going to do. Position her on her affected side, so the drainage won't contaminate her other eye.

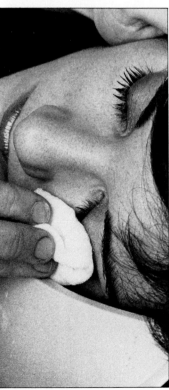

2 Moisten a sterile gauze pad with sterile normal saline solution. Then, gently clean any crusts or secretions from the patient's eyelids. *Remember:* Always wipe from the inner to the outer canthus to prevent contamination.

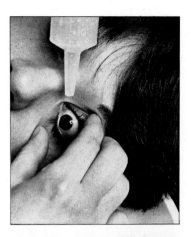

3 Use your thumb and index finger to open the patient's eyelids. With the fingers of your other hand, gently squeeze the bottle or bulb to direct a stream of irrigating solution into her eye. Be sure to start at the inner canthus, like the nurse is doing here. Don't start at the outer canthus, or you may spill the solution into the patient's other eye, contaminating it. To further prevent contamination, avoid touching the patient's eye or eyelids with the irrigator's tip.

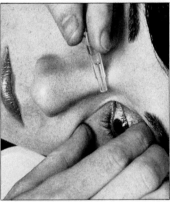

4 Suppose you'll need a large quantity of irrigating solution; for example, if your patient has a chemical burn. Prepare a 1,000 ml bottle of the prescribed solution, making sure it's room temperature. Attach I.V. tubing to the bottle. Then, direct the solution into the patient's eye, using a flow clamp to adjust the stream.

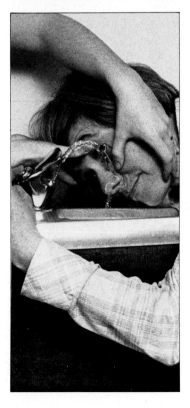

5 In an emergency, don't waste precious time gathering the irrigation equipment. Instead, take the patient to the nearest water faucet or water fountain. Adjust the water temperature to lukewarm, and make sure the flow's not too forceful. Then, position the patient so her affected eye is directly under the running water. Flush her eye for *at least 15 minutes*. Then, notify the doctor immediately.

When you've finished the irrigation, gently dry the patient's eyelids and cheek with gauze or cotton. Discard the drainage, and document the entire procedure on your patient's chart.

EENT emergencies

How to apply eye patches

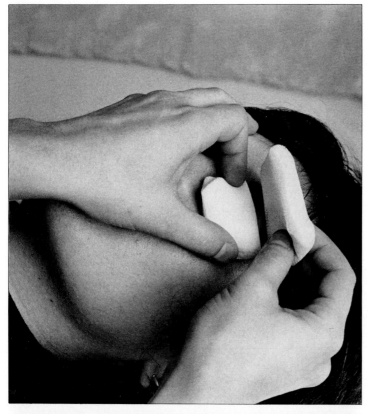

1 *Does the doctor want your patient to have one or both eyes patched? To find out how to apply eye patches correctly, read the following photostory.*

Before you begin, ask your patient to close *both* eyes. She may have difficulty closing only one. Place the patch over the affected eye.

Is the patch thick enough to fill the orbital depth? If not, you'll need to build up several layers, so the patch comes above the eye's bony orbital rim. To do so, fold one patch in half to create a base; then, add the other layers, creating just enough pressure to keep the eye closed.

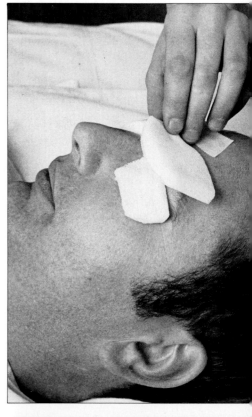

2 Now, as shown here, secure the patch with cellophane or paper tape.

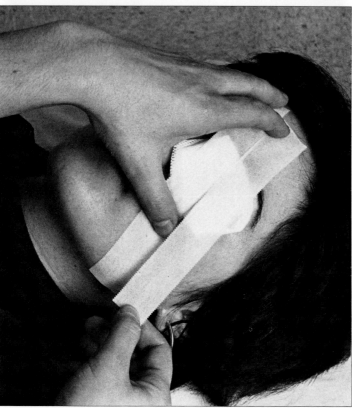

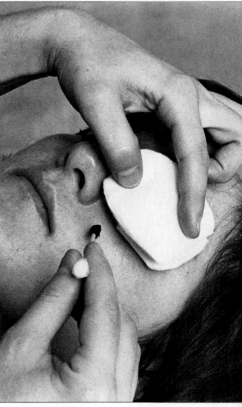

3 If your patient has a condition that affects both eyes, or if he's unconscious and can't close his eyes completely, he'll need both eyes patched. As you know, faulty closure will interfere with the eyes' natural lubrication and possibly lead to serious corneal damage. To prevent damage, gently close each eye, and apply a patch moistened with normal saline solution. Or put antibiotic ointment in the patient's eye, and cover it with a dry patch. Tape as before. Be sure to check the dressings periodically, and change them as the doctor orders.

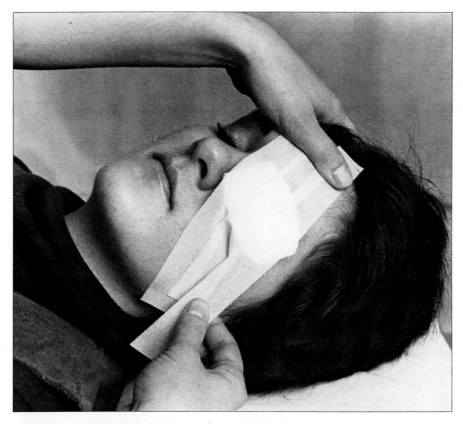

4 The doctor may order a pressure dressing for your patient's eye, to minimize eye movement and prevent post-traumatic edema. Do you know how to apply such a dressing? Have the patient sit up, if possible, with her eyes closed. Place an extra thick layer of patches over her affected eye, about twice as thick as for a regular patch. Make sure you cover the patient's eyebrow, so it will be protected from the adhesive tape that you'll apply later. Then, coat her cheek and forehead with tincture of benzoin to help the tape adhere better and prevent skin irritation.

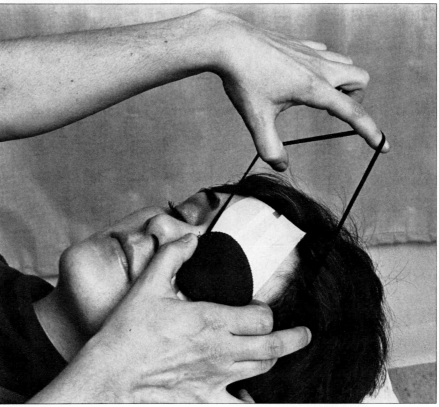

5 Next, apply several strips of non-allergenic tape diagonally across the patch, as shown here. Notice how the tape extends all the way from the patient's jawline to the opposite side of her forehead.

Sometimes, a patient with a pressure dressing on one eye will have swelling and discoloration around her unaffected eye. This may occur because the pressure dressing has caused a fluid shift from the damaged to the undamaged eye. Notify the doctor immediately.

6 Along with the eye patch, the doctor may also want your patient to have an eye shield. To apply, fit the shield over your patient's eye, and slip the elastic strap around her head. An eye shield may also help a patient who is light sensitive or has a corneal abrasion.

Remember: An eye patch or shield will decrease the patient's peripheral vision. Make sure you help the patient overcome any difficulties she has adjusting to this. Also, remind her not to drive a car or operate dangerous equipment.

EENT emergencies

Inspecting your patient's ear

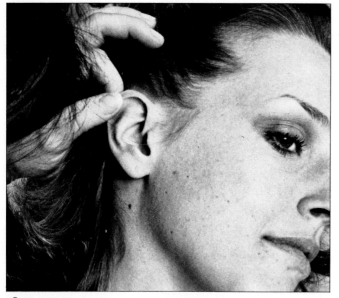

1 *Caring for a patient with an ear injury or infection? If so, you may have to inspect her ears. Here's how:*
First, place your patient in a seated position. Tilt her head away from you so you can better see inside the affected ear. Now, look at the external auditory canal. If a foreign body is visible, remove it by carefully grasping the object with a tweezers. *Note:* Removing porous or impacted matter from a patient's ear requires skill. If you have difficulty, notify the doctor at once.

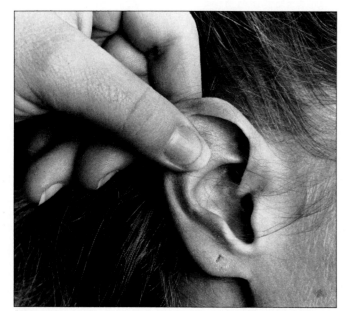

2 Next, straighten your patient's ear canal as much as possible. Do so by gently pulling the auricle upward and backward for an adult, or downward and backward for a child. Once the ear canal's properly positioned, begin examining the ear with an otoscope. For more information on how to use an otoscope, see the NURSING PHOTOBOOK *Assessing Your Patients.*

How to irrigate your patient's ear

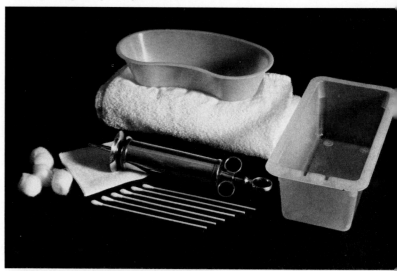

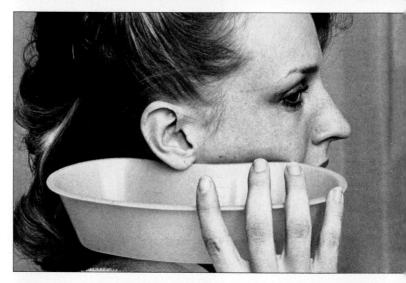

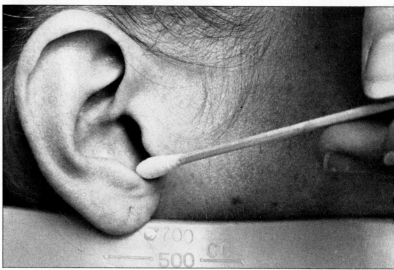

1 *Suppose the doctor orders an ear irrigation for your patient. Will you know what to do? You'll get the guidelines you need in this photostory.*

First, find out if the patient's ever had ear drainage, eardrum perforation, ear surgery, or any problems caused by a previous ear irrigation. (If she has, consult the doctor before proceeding.) Then, gather the following: a container of the prescribed irrigating solution, a bowl to pour it in, an ear syringe or plastic irrigation bottle, an emesis basin, cotton balls and applicators, towels, and a waste container. *Important:* Make sure the irrigating solution has been warmed to 100° F. (37.8° C.) before you proceed.

2 Explain the procedure to your patient and reassure her.

Then, have her sit or lie down, with her head tilted slightly toward the affected ear. Place towels around her shoulder area and—if she's able—ask her to hold the emesis basin under her ear.

Important: If your patient's a young child or mentally handicapped, the doctor may want her anesthetized. In such cases, the doctor will perform the irrigation.

3 Now, test the temperature of the irrigating solution by letting some of it flow over your inner arm. When you're sure it's okay, use a cotton applicator to check any outer ear discharge. Don't irrigate the patient's ear if you suspect she has *porous* foreign matter embedded in it. If you do, the foreign matter may expand and become even more firmly impacted.

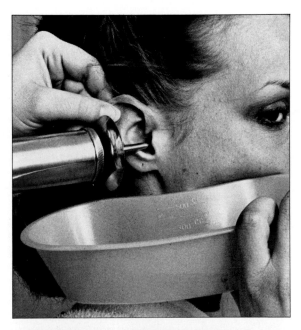

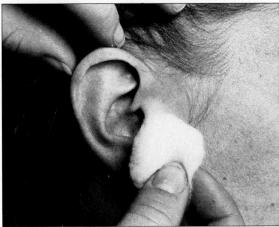

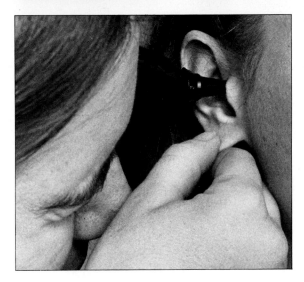

4 Straighten the ear canal, as described on the opposite page. Then, place the syringe tip or irrigating catheter at the entrance to the ear. Carefully direct a steady stream of irrigating solution toward the side of the ear canal. Be sure the fluid pressure's not too forceful, or you may damage the patient's eardrum.

As the returned fluid collects in the basin, watch it for cloudiness, cerumen, blood, or foreign matter. Continue the procedure until you've achieved the desired result, but don't use more than the allotted amount of solution (usually about 500 ml). *Important:* If your patient develops dizziness or pain, stop the irrigating procedure immediately.

5 Finally, dry your patient's ear with cotton balls, as shown here. Remove soiled towels, and make your patient comfortable.

If the irrigation's proved unsuccessful, instruct her to instill the ear medication ordered by the doctor. Then, tell her to return to her doctor or the ED for a repeat irrigation, if necessary.

Remember: Always document when you performed the ear irrigation, the kind and amount of solution used, your observations about the returned fluid, and the treatment's effect.

6 To determine the treatment's effectiveness, reinspect your patient's ear with an otoscope. For details on how to use an otoscope, see the NURSING PHOTOBOOK *Assessing Your Patients.*

EENT emergencies

When your patient needs an anterior/posterior nasal pack

1 *When the usual measures fail to control a patient's nosebleed, the doctor may insert an anterior/posterior nasal pack. Will you be ready to assist?*

First, gather the equipment shown in this photo: two #14 or #16 French catheters (get a smaller size if the patient is a child); 4" x 4" sterile gauze pads, three 18" (46 cm) silk sutures, two dental rolls, a bayonet forceps, a Kelly clamp, ½" Iodoform or Vaseline gauze, antibiotic ointment, lubricating jelly, nonallergenic tape, and a tongue depressor.

To make the posterior pack, roll a 4" x 4" sterile gauze pad, and cut it to the ordered size. Then, tie it together with three 18" (46 cm) silk sutures, as shown here. Leave a long end on each suture. You'll need these later when the pack's inserted.

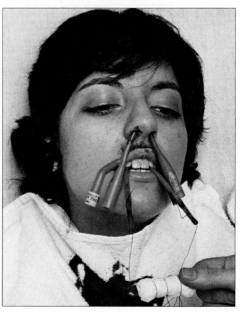

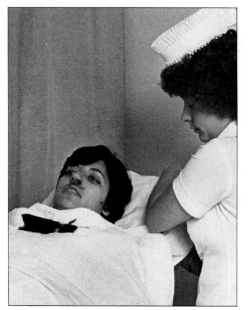

2 Now, reassure your patient, and explain the procedure. Place her in a seated position, if possible, or in a high Fowler's position on a stretcher or bed. Most likely the doctor will want you to administer a sedative. But remember, if your patient's lost a large amount of blood, the doctor may *not* want her to have a sedative. Why? Because it may mask signs of impending hypovolemic shock and may slow her respirations.

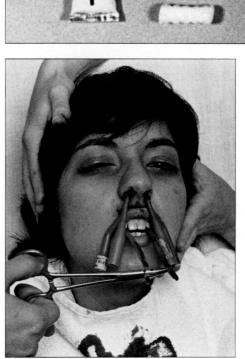

3 When the patient's prepared, the doctor will anesthetize her nasal passages with Xylocaine or a cocaine spray. Then, he'll insert one or both catheters into the patient's nostrils and slowly advance them to the nasopharynx. *Nursing tip:* Chances are the patient will gag during this part of the procedure. To minimize such discomfort, instruct her to pant.

As soon as the catheters are visible in the nasopharynx, the doctor will use a Kelly clamp, as shown here, to pull them out through her mouth.

4 Now, tie the posterior pack to the catheters, as shown here. To do this properly, use only the long sutures at each end of the pack. Let the middle suture hang free. Coat the entire pack with antibiotic ointment to minimize the risk of infection and to control odor.

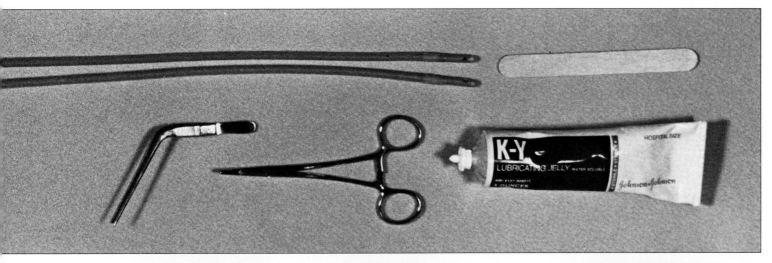

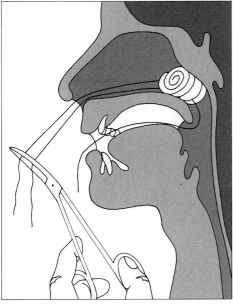

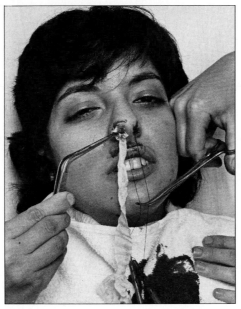

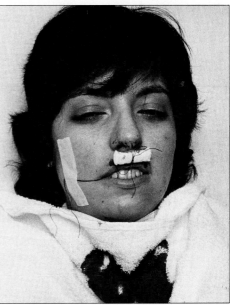

5 Stand by as the doctor pulls the posterior pack into place, above the patient's soft palate. He'll accomplish this by carefully withdrawing the catheters from the patient's nose.

When the pack's in place, examine the patient's throat to make sure her uvula isn't forced up underneath the pack. If all's well, use a Kelly clamp to grasp the sutures hanging from the patient's nose. As you can see in this illustration, the middle suture extends from the patient's mouth.

6 Hold the sutures tightly as the doctor packs the patient's nostrils with Iodoform or Vaseline gauze. Continue to reassure the patient. Remember, she'll probably be frightened and uncomfortable.

7 When the anterior pack's in place, tie the sutures extending from the patient's nose around a dental roll, as shown here. This will provide support and keep the nasal septum from becoming irritated. To make sure the dental roll's secure, use double knots. Finally, grasp the middle suture (hanging from the patient's mouth), and tape it to her cheek with nonallergenic tape.

Keep in mind that your patient can no longer breathe through her nose. If she starts to panic, do your best to calm her. Instruct her to breathe through her mouth while the pack's in place.

The doctor will want your patient to remain in the hospital for about 5 days. Document the entire procedure before you transfer her to another unit.

EENT emergencies

Nurses' guide to common EENT emergencies

Problem	Signs and symptoms	
Corneal abrasion, corneal ulcer	• Severe eye pain • Excessive tearing • Reddened conjunctiva	• Squinting • Photophobia • History of eye trauma or eye infection
Actinic trauma (welder's flash)	• History of overexposure to sunlight, ultraviolet light source (sunlamp), welding arc, or germicidal lamp	• Severe eye pain that may begin several hours after exposure
Laceration of the eyeball	• Severe eye pain; poor vision • External leakage of ocular fluid • Embedded foreign body	• Blood in anterior chamber of eye • History of recent blow to the eye or an injury to surrounding tissue
Contusion of the eyeball	• Eye pain; poor vision • History of recent blow to eye or injury to surrounding tissue (black eye)	• Patient complains of blurred vision, spots, or light flashes (all signs of possible retinal detachment)
Perforated eardrum	• Severe ear pain, possibly followed by a sudden decrease in pain as the eardrum ruptures • Ear drainage	• Fever • Possible bleeding • Burns in or surrounding ear
Epistaxis	• Frank bleeding from nose • Restlessness; anxiety; apprehension; cool, clammy skin; rapid, thready pulse; low blood pressure (all signs of hypovolemic shock) • Pale mucous membranes in nasal passages	• Patient lives or works in hot, unhumidified environment. Has history of nasal injury, recent upper respiratory infection, hypertension, blood dyscrasia, coronary artery disease, or alcoholism.
Fractured tooth	• If tooth enamel is involved, the fracture site will be rough but not sensitive to touch. • If the dentin is exposed, the tooth may be sensitive to touch or air. The color of the fracture surface will be yellowish-brown.	• If the fracture has exposed the pulp, the tooth will appear pink. It will be painful when tooth is touched. • If the root is involved, the tooth will be loose. It will be painful when tooth is touched.
Fractured larynx	• Severe face and neck pain • Anterior cervical neck area appears flat • Subcutaneous emphysema over larynx	• Nonpalpable thyroid cartilage • Dysphagia and hoarseness
Acute epiglottitis	• Dyspnea or apnea in severe cases • High fever • Inspiratory stridor in children (rarely heard in adults)	• Severe sore throat, with cherry-red, enlarged epiglottis • Possible substernal retraction on inspiration • Coughing and hoarseness
Hemorrhage post-tonsillectomy or postadenoidectomy	• Signs of hypovolemic shock: restlessness; agitation; diaphoresis; apprehension; rapid, thready pulse; low blood pressure; and cool, clammy skin	• Frank bleeding from mouth

Emergency nursing considerations

• If your patient's pain is so severe he can't tolerate an adequate eye examination, administer a topical anesthetic to his affected eye. Be sure to get a doctor's order before you do. Or check your hospital's policy on such things. *Important:* Before administering medication, make sure your patient's not allergic to it. Also, take care not to use an outdated medication.
• Examine the affected eye with a flashlight. If no lesion's visible but you strongly suspect one, call the doctor. He may instill fluorescein sodium (Ful-Glo Strips*) and examine the eye under a slit lamp or ultraviolet light. Irrigate your patient's eye with artificial tears after the exam.

• If examination reveals a corneal abrasion or ulcer, the doctor may ask you to instill antibiotic ointment and apply an eye patch. (For details on how to apply an eye patch, see pages 60 and 61.)
• Apply warm compresses to the affected eye, if ordered, to help relieve discomfort. Be sure your patient's eye is closed *before* you apply a compress to it.
• Give oral medication for pain, if ordered.
• To help relieve photophobia, instruct your patient to wear dark glasses.

• Instill anesthetic eye drops, antibiotic ointment, or antibiotic eye drops in affected eye, as ordered. Apply patches to both eyes. (For details, see page 60.) *Note:* The doctor may order eye patches to remain in place for 24 hours. Make sure your patient can get home safely and won't be left alone during the 24-hour period.

• Give analgesic, as ordered. Reassure your patient that his eye pain probably won't last longer than 24 hours.
• Instruct your patient to see an ophthalmologist for a follow-up examination, if pain persists. Otherwise, your patient can remove the eye patches and resume normal activities.

• Call the doctor immediately.
• Reassure your patient, and instruct him to lie flat until the doctor arrives. Meanwhile, apply an eye shield to help protect the affected eye. Don't permit the shield to press on the eyeball.
• Get a detailed history of the injury. Include the time of the accident, as well as how it occurred.

• Avoid touching the patient's eye during the examination. Use very *light pressure,* or you'll cause further injury.
• Administer a sedative, as ordered, and prepare your patient for surgery, if his condition requires it.

• Call the doctor immediately.
• *Caution:* During eye examination, don't touch the patient's eye more than once, especially if it feels soft.
• Reassure your patient, and have him lie on his back, with his head elevated on a small pillow. Then, cover the affected eye with an eye shield, and apply an ice pack.
• Get a detailed history of the injury.

• If the injury's minor, the doctor may want an ice pack applied to the affected eye for the first 24 hours, then warm compresses every 15 minutes thereafter. Instruct your patient how to apply warm compresses, and explain their importance.
• Administer a sedative, as ordered, and prepare your patient for surgery, if his condition requires it.

• Reassure your patient. Have an otoscope ready, and assist the doctor with ear exam.
• Get patient's complete medical history.
• If perforation is caused by penetrating object, have tweezers available to remove any imbedded particles. Never irrigate the ear.

• If burns are present, give burn care as needed.
• Give antibiotic ear drops, as ordered.
• Instruct your patient to keep his ear clean and dry. Tell him to place a cotton ball or ear mold inside his outer ear when showering or shampooing.

• Get the patient's medical history. Find out if he's taking any medications for recent illness. Look for Medic Alert bracelet to see if patient has blood dyscrasia.
• If patient has a blood dyscrasia, the doctor may want you to administer vitamin K₁* and plasma.
• Place patient in seated position. Instruct him to pinch his nose shut with 4" x 4" sterile gauze pads. Bend his head forward slightly so he won't swallow any blood. If that's unsuccessful, apply ice to back of his neck.

• Be ready to assist the doctor as he examines the patient's nose. Have necessary equipment on hand: a nasal speculum; a suction device, with angulated nasal tip; cocaine strips; electrocautery apparatus; silver nitrate sticks; and leads from chromic acid beads.
• If the doctor can't stop the bleeding, he may want you to help insert an anterior or anterior/posterior nasal pack. (To find out how, see pages 64 and 65.) The doctor may also choose to use this method if the patient has a blood dyscrasia.

• Gather the following equipment: dental burs, stone or sandpaper disks. The doctor may need these to smooth jagged tooth edges.
• If dentin is involved, cover the fractured area with a clean 2" x 2" sterile gauze pad. Administer pain medication, as ordered, while patient waits for the dentist.

• If pulp is exposed, place a sedative dressing on the exposed area, per doctor's order. Prepare for dentist to perform partial pulpotomy or pulpectomy, if necessary.
• If the root is involved, the doctor may want you to give the patient a pain medication. Prepare patient for possible tooth extraction by dentist.

• Don't leave patient. Reassure him.
• Be alert for possible airway obstruction. Have trach set and suction equipment ready. Doctor may perform bedside tracheotomy.

• Always look for laryngeal trauma or fracture in a patient with multiple injuries. Remember, a halter seat belt can cause fractured larynx in a car accident victim.

• Make sure patient has an open airway. If he's in a seated position, thrust his chest forward and hyperextend his neck.
• Be prepared to assist doctor if he wants to intubate patient or do an emergency tracheotomy.

• Be prepared to start appropriate I.V. therapy with antibiotics and steroids, per doctor's orders.

• Keep patient calm.
• After tonsillectomy, depress tongue sufficiently with tongue blade to examine pharynx. Look for blood clot, which may mask posterior bleeding into stomach.

• If patient shows signs of shock, start an I.V. with appropriate solution and draw a blood sample for type and crossmatching.
• Gather the following equipment for the doctor: electrocautery apparatus, sutures, and posterior packs.

---

*Available in the United States and in Canada.

Cardiopulmonary emergencies

Do you know what to do for a patient with severe chest injuries? How quickly and efficiently you respond may make the difference between whether he lives or dies. Consider your skills. Test them by asking yourself the following questions:

• How do you recognize and support a flail chest?

• What do you do first when the patient has a sucking chest wound?

• How do you assist the doctor when the patient needs a chest tube?

If you're not sure exactly what to do in emergencies of this type, pay special attention to the information that follows. The procedures illustrated and photographed on these pages will provide you with the knowledge necessary to perfect your skills.

Common thoracic injuries: Recognizing signs and symptoms

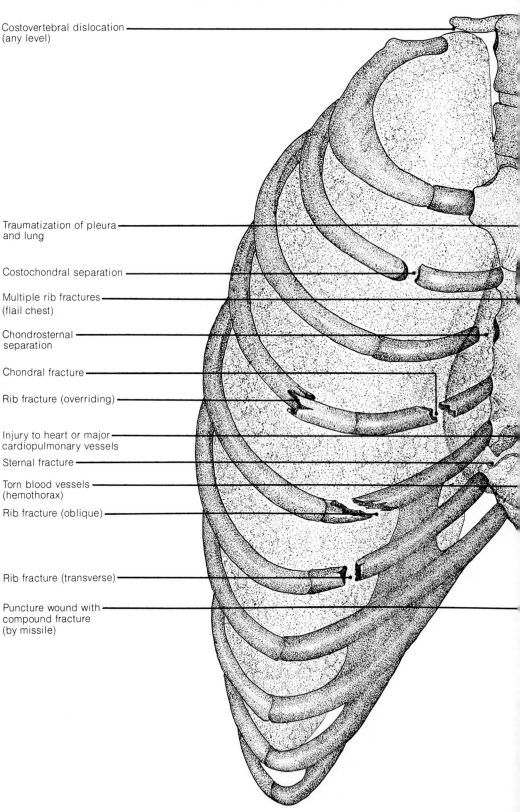

Costovertebral dislocation (any level)

Traumatization of pleura and lung

Costochondral separation

Multiple rib fractures (flail chest)

Chondrosternal separation

Chondral fracture

Rib fracture (overriding)

Injury to heart or major cardiopulmonary vessels

Sternal fracture

Torn blood vessels (hemothorax)

Rib fracture (oblique)

Rib fracture (transverse)

Puncture wound with compound fracture (by missile)

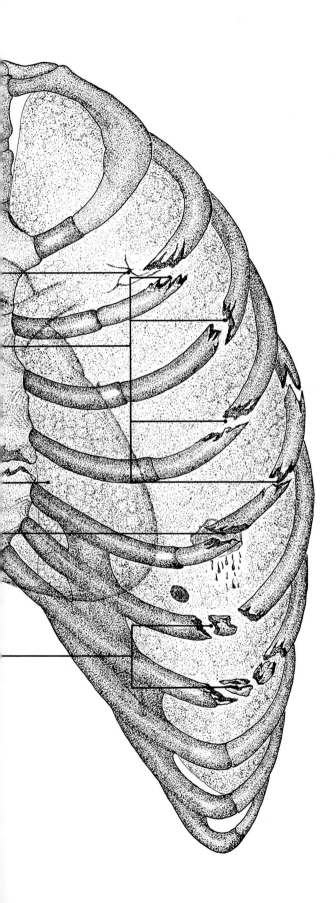

Many of the thoracic injuries you'll encounter in the emergency department are illustrated here. Study the information included with this drawing carefully. By familiarizing yourself with the signs and symptoms of these injuries now, you'll be better able to recognize and care for such patients later.

Costochondral or chondrosternal separation, or costovertebral dislocation
Suspect it when the patient has history of direct anterior impact to chest; on palpation, localized tenderness; "clicking" sensation during respiration.

Trauma to pleura and/or lung (for example, pneumothorax, lung contusion)
Suspect it when the patient has history of recent blunt chest injury, chest pain, shortness of breath, distant or absent breath sounds over injured area.

Multiple rib fractures (flail chest)
Suspect it when the patient has subcutaneous emphysema, pain at fracture site, tenderness on palpation, bone crepitus, paradoxical chest movement, respiratory difficulty.

Chondral or sternal fracture
Suspect it when the patient has recent severe chest wall trauma; sharp, excruciating pain at the fracture site; subcutaneous emphysema; swelling and visible deformity over the fracture site; tenderness when sternum is palpated.

Rib fracture (overriding, oblique, transverse)
Suspect it when the patient has localized tenderness or subcutaneous emphysema over the injured site; difficult, painful respirations; paradoxical chest movement.

Injury to heart or major cardiopulmonary vessels
Suspect it when the patient has ecchymotic areas over chest wall, cardiac arrhythmia, palpitations or precordial pain, cough, nausea, and vomiting.

Torn blood vessels (hemothorax)
Suspect it when the patient has history of recent blunt chest trauma, hypotension, respiratory distress, tightness in chest, mediastinal shift on X-ray, signs of shock with severe bleeding.

Puncture wound
Suspect it when the patient has signs of severe respiratory distress, sucking sound during respiration, subcutaneous emphysema, visible lung through puncture.

Esophageal injury (not shown)
Suspect it when the patient has dyspnea, cyanosis, upper abdominal pain, hypotension, subcutaneous emphysema in cervical or anterior thoracic regions, signs and symptoms identical to tracheobronchial disruption that can't be attributed to tracheobronchial damage.

Tracheobronchial disruption (not shown)
Suspect it when the patient has dyspnea, hemoptysis, subcutaneous emphysema, cyanosis.

Ruptured diaphragm (not shown)
Suspect it when the patient has history of recent chest or abdominal trauma; marked respiratory distress; cyanosis; hypotension; bowel sounds heard in thorax; pain in abdomen (usually left upper quadrant), left lower thorax, or left shoulder.

Cardiopulmonary emergencies

Nurses' guide to cardiopulmonary emergencies

Do you know what emergency care to give in the following cardiopulmonary emergencies? The chart below will give you specific instructions. Study them carefully. In addition, remember these guidelines that apply to every cardiopulmonary emergency:

Call the doctor immediately. Make sure the patient has an open airway. Monitor him closely for signs of shock, and begin I.V. therapy, as needed, with the appropriate solution. Draw blood for type and crossmatching in case your patient needs a blood transfusion. Get a complete medical history from the patient or his family, including information about the accident or injury (when applicable).

Problem	Signs and symptoms	Special emergency nursing considerations
Cardiac contusion	• History of injury to anterior chest • Ecchymosis on chest wall • Retrosternal angina, unrelieved by nitroglycerin, but sometimes relieved by O₂ therapy • Tachycardia • EKG reading indicating *apparent* myocardial infarction or conduction disturbances • Pericardial friction rub • *Important:* In some cases, a patient with a cardiac contusion may be completely asymptomatic.	• Follow the general guidelines listed above. • Stay alert for signs of a ruptured aorta or ventricle which may develop from this condition. Also watch for signs of cardiac tamponade. (You'll find complete details later in this chart.) • Prepare patient for admission to the hospital. The doctor will want him to have continuous EKG monitoring.
Penetrating wound in heart	• In most cases, patient has a visible chest wound, caused by object like knife or bullet. However, heart penetration can occur from a bullet entering the abdomen or back. • Chest pain, bleeding • Drowsiness, loss of consciousness, possible agitation, combativeness, or confusion. (Note: Patient may appear intoxicated.) • Tachycardia, muffled heart sounds, hypotension, dyspnea, increased central venous pressure (CVP), possible cardiac arrest • Distended neck veins, although these may not be present immediately. For example, if the patient's in hypovolemic shock from blood loss, he may not have neck vein distention until he receives adequate I.V. fluid replacement. • Pneumothorax or hemothorax. (May not develop until several hours after the injury.)	• Follow the general guidelines listed above. • If a penetrating object, like a knife, is still in place when the patient arrives in the ED, don't remove it. Let it act as a seal for the damaged blood vessels and heart. (For further information on how to care for such wounds, see page 73.) • Place patient on cardiac monitor. • If the penetrating object's already been removed, control bleeding by applying direct pressure to the wound with a sterile cloth. • Administer oxygen. Be prepared to intubate the patient, if necessary. • If the doctor decides to insert a chest tube, be ready to assist. (For full details, see the NURSING PHOTOBOOK *Providing Respiratory Care.* • Prepare patient for a thoracotomy.
Cardiac tamponade (a condition in which fluid, blood, or blood clots become trapped between the heart muscle and the pericardial sac or anterior chest wall)	• History of cardiac contusion, blunt trauma to anterior chest, penetrating chest wound, or recent cardiac surgery. *Important:* Cardiac tamponade may also be a complication of an existing medical problem; for example, infectious pericardial neoplasm, or uremia. In addition, tamponade may follow these procedures: cardiac catheterization or pacemaker insertion (from perforation of right heart ventricle), CPR, or diagnostic pericardial tap. • Dyspnea, possible cyanosis, agitation, and neck vein distention • Weak, thready pulse or paradoxical pulse in which blood pressure drops on inspiration • Absent third heart sound • Hypotension with narrowed pulse pressure • Increased central venous pressure (CVP) • Decreased urinary output	• Follow the general guidelines listed above. • Prepare to assist the doctor with a pericardiocentesis. Assemble the following equipment: pericardiocentesis tray, crash cart, I.V. fluids, endotracheal tubes, hand-held resuscitator, defibrillator, and cardiac pacemaker. • Place patient on cardiac monitor. • Administer oxygen. • Following pericardiocentesis, prepare patient for a thoracotomy. As you do, observe him closely for recurring signs of tamponade, which may result in cardiac arrest. • Watch for signs of pulmonary emboli: extreme agitation, dyspnea, pallor, combativeness, chest pain. Notify doctor immediately.

Problem	Signs and symptoms	Special emergency nursing considerations
Ruptured aorta	• History of abrupt deceleration or compression injury • Chest or back pain • Dyspnea; weak, thready pulse; weakness in extremities; drowsiness, loss of consciousness • In some cases, increased blood pressure and pulse amplitude in upper extremities, coupled with decreased blood pressure and pulse amplitude in lower extremities	• Follow the general guidelines listed on the opposite page. • Prepare patient for immediate surgery. • Administer oxygen, and place patient on cardiac monitor. • Have the following equipment nearby: tubes, hand-held resuscitator, and mechanical ventilator. • Get ready to administer nitroprusside (Nipride*), according to doctor's order. Remember to protect the container from light. • When you monitor patient's vital signs, pay particular attention to the pulses in his legs.
Pneumothorax (air in pleural space)	• History of blunt chest trauma caused by fall, blow, violent cough, or sudden deceleration • History of penetrating chest injury, such as a knife or bullet wound. May also be a complication caused by CVP line insertion or thoracentesis • Possible sudden, sharp chest pain, sometimes referred to shoulder, opposite side of chest, or abdomen • Dyspnea, dry hacking cough, diminished or absent breath sounds on affected side, asymmetric chest movements • Hyperresonance on percussion • Possible subcutaneous emphysema (crepitus) on neck or chest wall	• Follow the general guidelines listed on the opposite page. • If a patient has a penetrating chest wound, prepare to assist doctor with immediate insertion of flutter valve or chest tube. (To learn how to make a flutter valve, see the NURSING PHOTOBOOK *Providing Respiratory Care.* • If the patient needs oxygen, administer it with a nasal cannula or face mask, at 4 to 10 liters per minute. However, if your patient has chronic obstructive pulmonary disease (COPD), administer oxygen at 2 liters (or less) per minute. • Prepare to intubate the COPD patient, if necessary. • Watch for signs of mediastinal shift. (See information listed on page 72.)
Hemothorax (blood in pleural space)	• History of trauma to chest wall, lung tissue, or mediastinum; pleural or pulmonary neoplasm; pulmonary infarction; or pleural tear from spontaneous pneumothorax. May also be a complication of anticoagulant therapy after chest surgery. • Chest pain; dyspnea; tachycardia; diaphoresis; hypotension; skin color changes; asymmetric chest movements (if hemothorax is large); frothy or bloody sputum; weak, thready pulse; rapid, shallow respirations; possible cyanosis; EKG changes; and ecchymosis over affected area • Diminished or absent breath sounds on affected side; dullness on percussion • Possible rib or sternum fracture	• Follow the general guidelines listed on the opposite page. • Administer oxygen by nasal cannula or mask. • Be prepared to assist doctor with chest tube insertion. After the chest tube's inserted, record the initial amount of bloody drainage on the patient's chart. If it exceeds 1,000 ml, prepare patient for an immediate thoracotomy. If bloody drainage is less than 1,000 ml, continue caring for patient as before. Monitor drainage amount carefully. Notify doctor immediately if drainage exceeds 500 ml within the first 3 hours. • Draw an arterial blood sample to obtain blood gas measurements.

*Available in the United States and in Canada.

Cardiopulmonary emergencies

Nurses' guide to cardiopulmonary emergencies continued

Problem	Signs and symptoms	Special emergency nursing considerations
Mediastinal shift 	• History of tension pneumothorax • Displacement of trachea and larynx from middle toward unaffected side • Chest assessment reveals displaced cardiac dullness, shift in apex beat, and cardiac arrhythmias • Neck vein distention • Severe hypotension	• Follow the general guidelines listed on page 70. • Place patient on cardiac monitor. • Prepare to assist doctor immediately with insertion of flutter valve or chest tube.
Pulmonary contusion 	• History of blunt trauma to lung (usually caused by high-velocity impact)	• Follow the general guidelines listed on page 70. • Administer oxygen immediately, even if patient is asymptomatic. Hypoxemia may develop rapidly. • Place patient in high Fowler's position to help ease breathing efforts. • Prepare to place patient on mechanical ventilation, if necessary. • Draw arterial blood sample to obtain blood gas measurements. • Prepare patient for chest X-rays. • Place patient on cardiac monitor. • If the patient's lost a large amount of blood, the doctor may decide to do an emergency thoracotomy. Be prepared to assist him.
Ruptured diaphragm 	• History of blunt trauma (usually one-sided) or multiple trauma (especially involving fractured pelvis) • Severe chest pain or referred pain in abdomen or shoulder; dyspnea and cyanosis; chest assessment reveals decreased or absent breath sounds on affected side; and dullness, tympany, or bowel sounds on affected side from herniated viscera • Possible mediastinal or tracheal shift away from affected side • *Important:* In some cases, patient may be asymptomatic.	• Follow the general guidelines listed on page 70. • Carefully examine and evaluate entrance and exit wounds. The diaphragm's position at the time of the accident will determine the extent of injury. For example, a bullet that enters on the anterior *right* side of the patient's rib cage (above the costal margin) and exits on the posterior right side (at the 10th-rib level) will involve the patient's liver. A similar injury on the patient's *left* side will involve his spleen, stomach, colon, and small bowel. • Administer oxygen, as ordered. Prepare to intubate patient, if necessary, and use mechanical ventilation. • Place patient on cardiac monitor. • Insert nasogastric tube to prevent possible respiratory and circulatory impairment from herniated abdominal viscera. If ordered, use suction or administer an iced saline solution lavage to relieve gastric bleeding. • If the patient's lung has been punctured, get ready to assist the doctor with chest tube insertion. • Prepare patient for surgery, if necessary.

How to manage a sucking chest wound

1 *Late one night, 35-year-old Vince DeSantos is accidentally knifed in a domestic quarrel and is brought to the ED with the weapon still embedded in his chest. Your ears tell you he has a sucking chest wound, so you act quickly.*

As you know, sucking chest wounds are life-threatening, because they destroy the necessary pressure gradient between the pleural space and outside atmosphere. Unless you can restore this pressure gradient, the patient will quickly go into respiratory failure.

Here's what to do: First, make sure the patient is receiving oxygen, as shown in this photo.

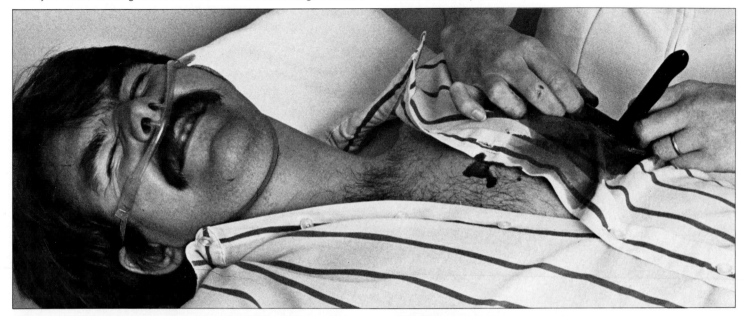

2 *Don't remove the knife.* Never remove any object penetrating a patient's chest, either in the ED or at the accident scene. Doing so will destroy the pressure gradient even faster and increase bleeding. First, reassure Mr. DeSantos and ask for his cooperation. Instruct him to exhale forcefully. At the moment of maximum expiration, seal the wound closed by covering it with Vaseline gauze.

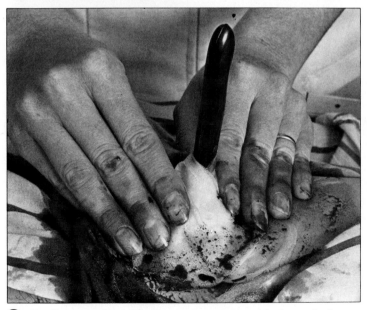

3 Secure the gauze with wide tape, as the nurse is doing in this photo. (If you don't have any Vaseline gauze handy, cover the wound with a towel until you or another nurse can get some.)

When you've covered the wound, watch the patient closely. If he starts developing signs of respiratory distress, suspect a tension pneumothorax, and remove the gauze immediately.

Prepare Mr. DeSantos for surgery, as ordered by the doctor. If the doctor decides to insert a chest tube before Mr. DeSantos is taken to the OR, gather the equipment you'll need, and get ready to assist.

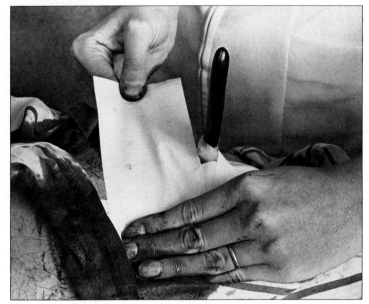

Cardiopulmonary emergencies

When your patient needs a chest tube: Your role

1 *Let's assume you're caring for 45-year-old John Whitaker when the doctor decides Mr. Whitaker needs a chest tube. Are you prepared to assist while he inserts it? Do you know how to assemble the equipment you need for chest drainage? Here's what to do:*

First, explain what's going to happen, and answer any questions Mr. Whitaker may have. Make sure he's signed the necessary surgical consent form. Then, gather the equipment the doctor will need (including a suction device), and obtain a disposable Pleur-evac®. Unwrap the Pleur-evac carefully, and set it on a disposable floor stand or hang it from the bedframe. To fill it, you'll need a large container of sterile water and a 60 cc piston or bulb syringe.

Note: Suppose a Pleur-evac's not available. Use a glass bottle underwater-seal chest drainage system instead. You'll find out exactly how to set it up in the NURSING PHOTOBOOK *Providing Respiratory Care.*

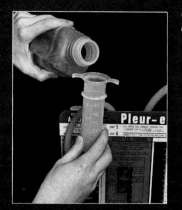

2 Next, remove the plastic connector on the short tube attached to the water-seal chamber of the Pleur-evac. Remove the plunger or bulb from the syringe and attach the barrel. Pour water into the tube, using the syringe barrel as a funnel.

Always fill the water-seal chamber to the 2 cm level, no matter what the doctor decides to do about suctioning. Check the water level periodically, and refill the chamber as needed.

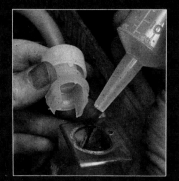

3 If the doctor decides suctioning won't be necessary, leave the end of the short tube unclamped. This will permit air to escape from the patient's pleural cavity. If the doctor *does* order suctioning, remove the plastic muffler from the vent to the suction control chamber. Then, attach a syringe barrel to the vent, using the same method as before, and pour water in the chamber.

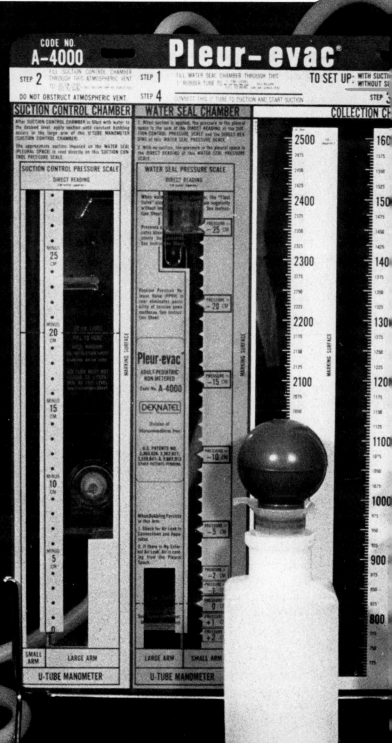

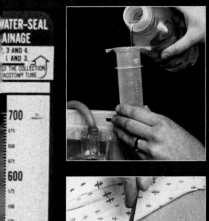

4 Fill the suction control chamber to the 20 cm level, or as ordered by the doctor. Replace the plastic muffler, to minimize the bubbling noise. Make sure nothing occludes the vent.

Important: Always check the water level in the suction chamber at least once each shift. If evaporation occurs, refill the chamber.

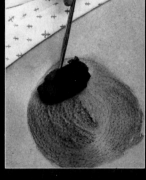

5 Now, position your patient correctly for chest tube insertion, according to the doctor's orders. In most cases, he'll probably want you to place the patient on his back. But he may want him lying on his side.

At this point, the doctor will cleanse the area he's chosen for the insertion and apply a local anesthetic, as shown here. Reassure the patient as the chest tube is inserted.

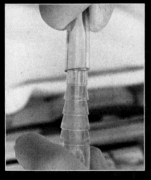

6 Now, remove the adapter from the long tube that extends from the Pleur-evac's collection chamber. Stand by as the doctor connects this tube to the patient's chest tube. Wrap the connections with adhesive tape to prevent air leaks and to keep the tubes together. However, never cover the plastic connector or you won't be able to observe the drainage.

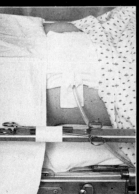

7 Whenever—or wherever—you care for a patient with a chest tube, be prepared for a situation in which you may have to clamp the tube; for example, if the Pleur-evac becomes disconnected. Keep two covered Kelly clamps nearby, where you can spot them quickly. (For complete details on how to clamp a patient's chest tube properly, see page 76.)

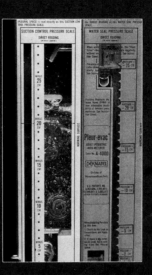

8 Has the doctor ordered suction? Connect the short tube on the water-seal chamber to the suction device, using the plastic connector provided. Turn on the suction, and slowly increase it until bubbling occurs in the suction control chamber.

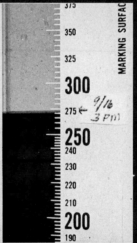

9 At the end of each shift, measure the drainage that's accumulated in the collection chamber. Record the date and time on a piece of tape, and attach it to the front of the Pleur-evac, at the drainage level. By doing this, you can assess further drainage quickly.

Remember: If the Pleur-evac's moved, drainage may spill into adjacent chambers. Always check the volume of each chamber before you total the output. Read all measurements at eye level.

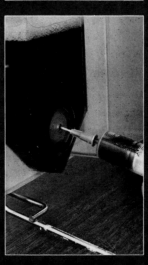

10 The doctor may order laboratory analysis of the chest drainage. Collect the specimen you need by inserting a syringe with an 18G or 20G needle into the self-sealing diaphragm in back of the collection chamber. Withdraw the desired amount, cap and label the syringe, and send it to the lab. Make sure the needle remains securely attached.

For more details on the care of patients requiring chest drainage, see the NURSING PHOTOBOOK *Providing Respiratory Care.*

Cardiopulmonary emergencies

How to clamp a chest tube

Suppose you're caring for a patient with a chest tube and the Pleur-evac becomes disconnected, or one of the glass drainage bottles breaks. You'll need to clamp the chest tube *immediately* and work quickly to correct the problem. Here's how:

• If your patient's conscious, tell him to cough or exhale forcefully.

• Take one of the covered Kelly clamps placed nearby (for such an emergency), and clamp the chest tube close to the chest wall. To make sure the tube's held securely, apply a second clamp pointed in the opposite direction (see photo below).

• Obtain a *new* Pleur-evac or glass drainage bottle immediately, and prepare to connect it. Never use the old Pleur-evac again; it may have become contaminated.

• Clean the chest tube with antiseptic solution before you connect it to the new drainage system. Unclamp the tube as soon as the connection is secure. Never leave a chest tube clamped for a prolonged period. Doing so could cause a tension pneumothorax.

Take immediate action to clamp the patient's chest tube in the situations described above. However, in the following situations, get a doctor's order for clamping:

• The drainage bottle or Pleur-evac becomes full and needs replacing.

• You need to collect a drainage specimen from the bottle.

• Your patient's being transported with glass bottles and you want to minimize the risk of breakage.

• Your patient's condition has so improved that he may no longer need a chest tube. In such a case, the doctor may want you to clamp the tube before he removes it to test the patient's reaction.

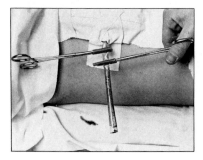

Supporting a flail chest

1 *Does your patient have multiple rib fractures? In most cases, rib fractures won't cause serious breathing difficulty, because the patient's chest wall will remain stable. However, if adjacent rib fractures occur in two or more places—causing a flail chest—the situation becomes life-threatening. Normal chest excursion will be lost, and the lung lying under the flail section won't expand and contract effectively. (To better understand exactly what happens, study this illustration.)*

Suspect flail chest in a patient with a crushing chest injury when he has severe pain, paradoxical chest movement, and dyspnea. Then, quickly follow the guidelines on the next page to prevent possible lung damage.

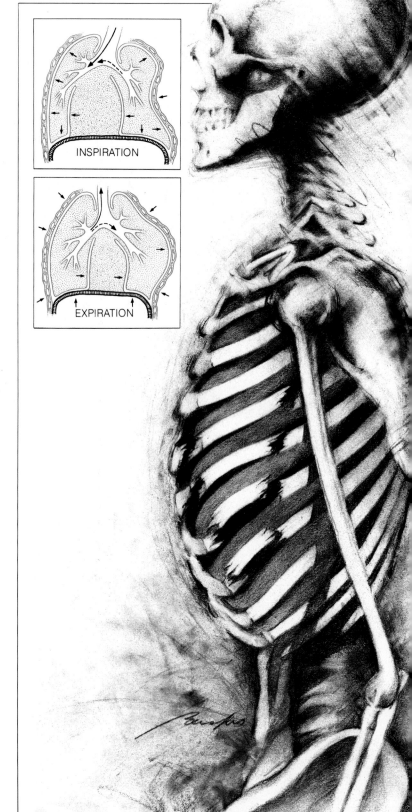

INSPIRATION

EXPIRATION

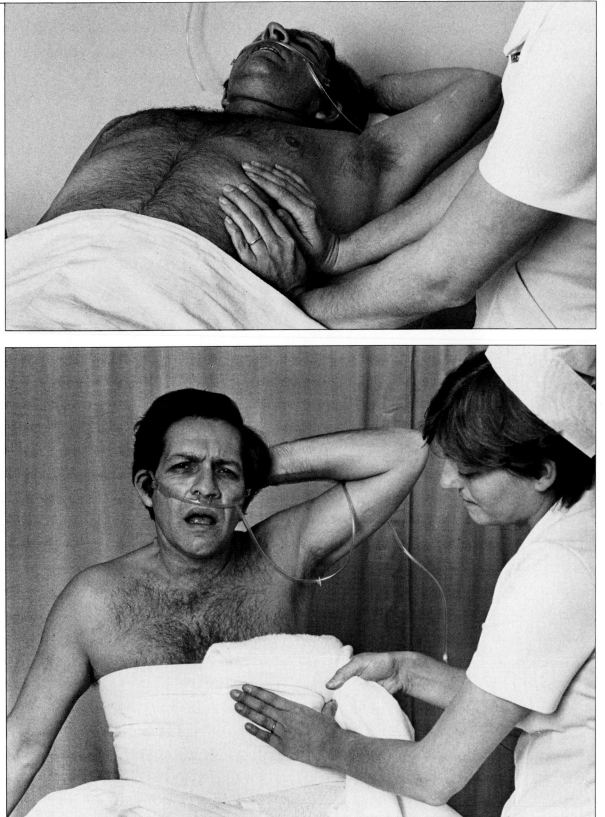

2 First, administer needed oxygen therapy. Then, stabilize the patient's chest wall by placing your hands over the flail site and applying pressure. If the patient also has an open wound in this area, apply pressure with a sterile towel or pad.

3 Or use a pillow or folded blanket to support the flail chest, as the nurse is doing here. Keep the pillow in place by wrapping the patient's entire chest area with a bed sheet.

Another way to support a flail chest is with a 10-pound (4.5 kg) sandbag. You could also position the patient on his affected side if you had to leave him momentarily to get help.

Whatever method you choose, reassure him by explaining the entire procedure. Remember, he'll no doubt be extremely anxious, especially if he's experiencing respiratory distress.

While the doctor determines how to repair the chest wall, continue giving emergency care. Make sure the patient's airway remains open. Use suctioning equipment, if necessary.

Abdominal/pelvic emergencies

How skilled are you at caring for a patient with abdominal/pelvic injuries? For example, do you know how and when to insert a Foley catheter? How to perform an emergency bladder irrigation? How to assist the doctor with a peritoneal lavage?

What about the internal complications that may develop from injuries in this area? Are you prepared to cope with them? Your advanced knowledge and skills are critical in such emergencies. They may help to save the patient's life.

Study the following pages carefully. You'll find them informative and helpful. They're packed with nursing tips that'll make your job easier. When you've reviewed everything in these photostories, refer to Section 4. It describes even more emergency conditions relating to the abdominal/pelvic area, and tells you what to do about them.

Assessing abdominal/pelvic injuries

When a patient comes to the ED with an abdominal or pelvic injury, consider which organs, major blood vessels, or bones may have been damaged. Doing so will help you know what to expect.

For example, suppose your patient has a fractured pelvis. The bone chips from such an injury could damage his bladder. Learn what complications can arise from specific injuries by studying the following pages. Use this illustration as a guide in your assessment.

Ruptured diaphragm —————

Contused or lacerated liver —————

Ruptured spleen —————

Avulsed adrenal —————

Contused or avulsed kidney —————

Perforated stomach —————

Ruptured gallbladder —————

Fractured pancreas —————

Lacerated, ruptured, or —————
transected bowel

Severed ureter —————

Lacerated or ruptured major
blood vessels: aorta and vena cava —

Perforated rectum —————

Perforated bladder —————

Fractured pelvis: bone
fragments may damage other —————
organs, especially bladder

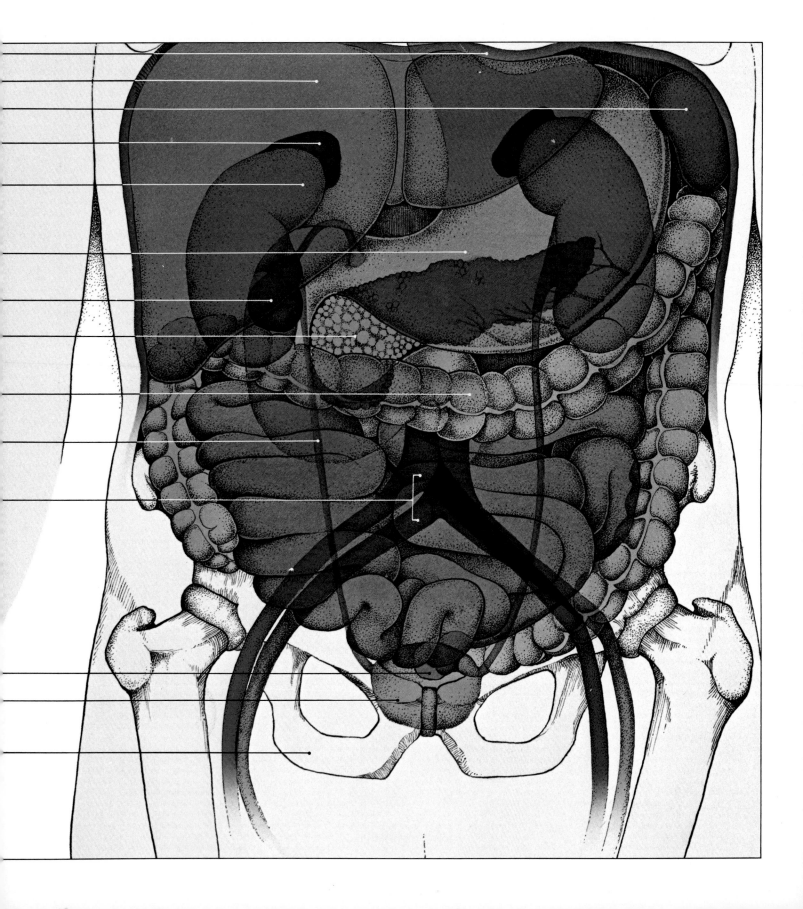

Abdominal/pelvic emergencies

Nurses' guide to abdominal/pelvic emergencies

Injury	Signs and symptoms	Special emergency nursing considerations	Possible associated injuries
Lacerated or fractured liver	• Pain in right upper abdominal quadrant • Signs of hypovolemic shock: rapid, thready pulse; low blood pressure; anxiety; restlessness; apprehension; decreased red blood cell count; elevated white blood cell count; cool, clammy skin; pallor • History of blunt or penetrating abdominal trauma	• If the doctor determines the patient has a large laceration or a fractured liver, he'll want you to prepare the patient for surgery. • If he determines the patient has a small tear, he may let it heal without further treatment. • Be ready to administer antibiotics, tetanus toxoid, as ordered by the doctor. • Continue to observe patient for signs and symptoms. • Be ready to assist doctor with peritoneal lavage (see page 83).	• Lacerated bowel • Right lower rib fractures • Avulsion of major hepatic vessels
Ruptured spleen	• Muscle spasm and rigidity in left upper abdominal quadrant • If diaphragm's irritated, the patient may have referred pain in his left shoulder and left upper abdominal quadrant (Kehr's sign). • If the patient's conscious, he may complain of abdominal tenderness. • Signs of hypovolemic shock, sometimes delayed (see above) • Enlarged spleen with medial displacement (evident in X-ray)	• Be ready to assist doctor with peritoneal lavage to confirm diagnosis. • Be ready to administer antibiotics, tetanus toxoid, as ordered by the doctor. • Prepare patient for possible arteriography. • Prepare patient for surgery.	• Left lower rib fractures • Stomach compression • Penetrating injuries of the stomach, pancreas, and bowel (splenic flexure)
Fractured pancreas	• Signs of hypovolemic shock (see above) • Mild epigastric tenderness. This pain occurs immediately after the injury, decreases over the next 2 hours, then worsens within 6 hours. • Absence of bowel sounds • Involuntary abdominal muscle spasm • Possible elevated serum amylase • History of blunt or penetrating abdominal trauma	• Be ready to administer antibiotics, tetanus toxoid, as ordered by the doctor. • Prepare patient for surgery.	• Crushed duodenum • Retroperitoneal cellulitis and abcess, pancreatic pseudocyst, and chronic recurrent pancreatitis may follow pancreatic fracture.
Perforated gastrointestinal tract	• Lower abdominal rigidity, with spasms • Appearance of blood in nasogastric fluid upon aspiration may indicate perforated stomach • Epigastric tenderness • History of penetrating trauma to upper abdomen or lower thorax	• Be ready to administer antibiotics, as ordered by the doctor. • Prepare patient for surgery. • Insert a nasogastric tube for aspiration of nasogastric contents (see pages 106 to 110).	• Lacerated duodenum, jejunum, and distal ileum • Small laceration of mesentery • Spillage of bowel contents into peritoneal cavity, with ensuing peritonitis • Perforated pancreas • Intramural hematoma • Liver or spleen injuries
Lacerated inferior vena cava	• Signs of hypovolemic shock (see above). *Note:* If your patient has retroperitoneal hematoma, he may not have signs of shock. • History of penetrating abdominal wound	• Control severe hemorrhage; apply a MAST suit, as ordered by the doctor. • Don't start an I.V. in the patient's leg, because the fluid may escape into his abdominal cavity. • Prepare patient for immediate surgery.	• Lacerated abdominal aorta or bowel • Retroperitoneal hematoma

Injury	Signs and symptoms	Special emergency nursing considerations	Possible associated injuries
Lacerated abdominal aorta	• Abdominal tenderness and rigidity • Signs of hypovolemic shock (see opposite page) • History of penetrating abdominal wound	• Don't start an I.V. in the patient's leg, because the fluid may escape into his abdominal cavity. • Prepare patient for immediate surgery.	• Lacerated inferior vena cava or bowel • Spinal cord injury
Urethral transection	• Gross bleeding or dried blood at urethral orifice • Perineal ecchymosis • Suprapubic pain • Difficult urination, accompanied by distended bladder; urge to urinate • If patient's a male, he may have upwardly displaced prostate.	• Instruct patient not to urinate. • Notify urologist. • Be prepared to assist urologist with insertion of suprapubic catheter. *Caution:* Don't insert a Foley catheter into the urethra. • Prepare patient for surgery.	• Perforated bladder • Rectal laceration
Fractured pelvis	• Signs of hypovolemic shock (see opposite page) • Pain in abdomen and back • Absent or diminished bowel sounds • Vomiting • Hematuria • Paralytic ileus • History of blunt abdominal/pelvic trauma	• Be prepared to insert a nasogastric tube. • Insert Foley catheter, as ordered by the doctor. • Stabilize patient's pelvis with a draw sheet or pillow. If available, apply a MAST suit, as indicated by the doctor, to reduce hemorrhage and counteract hypovolemia. • If ordered by the doctor, prepare patient for cystogram, to rule out bladder damage. • Prepare patient for abdominal/pelvic X-rays and/or arteriography. • Prepare patient for surgery. • After the patient's admitted, be ready to assist doctor with application of a pelvic sling.	• Perforated bladder or lower bowel • Urethral tears (more common in males) • Displaced prostate, surrounded by a collection of blood • Nerve damage, especially if the patient has a fractured sacrum • Lacerated uterus • Lacerated colon
Renal trauma	• Pain in midback or flank • Referred abdominal pain, which may worsen with movement • Hematuria (may be frank or occult) • Oliguria or anuria • Local ecchymosis, with possible edema • Local tenderness to the touch • History of penetrating thoracic, abdominal, or lower back trauma	• Insert a Foley catheter. • Be prepared to assist with a bladder irrigation. • Apply ice packs to reduce swelling. • Prepare patient for a possible cystogram, intravenous pyelogram (IVP), or renal arteriography, as ordered by the doctor. • After diagnostic tests are performed, administer analgesics, as ordered by the doctor. • In cases of severe trauma, prepare patient for surgery.	• Fractured pelvis
Perforated bladder	• Pain in lower abdominal or suprapubic area • Signs of hypovolemic shock (see opposite page) • Difficulty with bowel movement, accompanied by urge to void • Hematuria • Ecchymosis or bruising on lower abdomen, below the umbilicus • Large, suprapubic mass (possibly from a perivesical collection of urine and blood)	• Insert a Foley catheter to obtain urine specimen. • If urethral damage accompanies the bladder trauma, be prepared to assist the doctor with insertion of suprapubic catheter. • Prepare patient for a cystogram or an IVP, as ordered by the doctor. • Prepare patient for immediate surgery.	• Perforated peritoneum • Urethral damage

Abdominal/pelvic emergencies

Eight trouble indicators: What they suggest

Any of these conditions in a patient with an abdominal/pelvic injury may indicate a serious—perhaps life-threatening—situation. Notify the doctor at once.

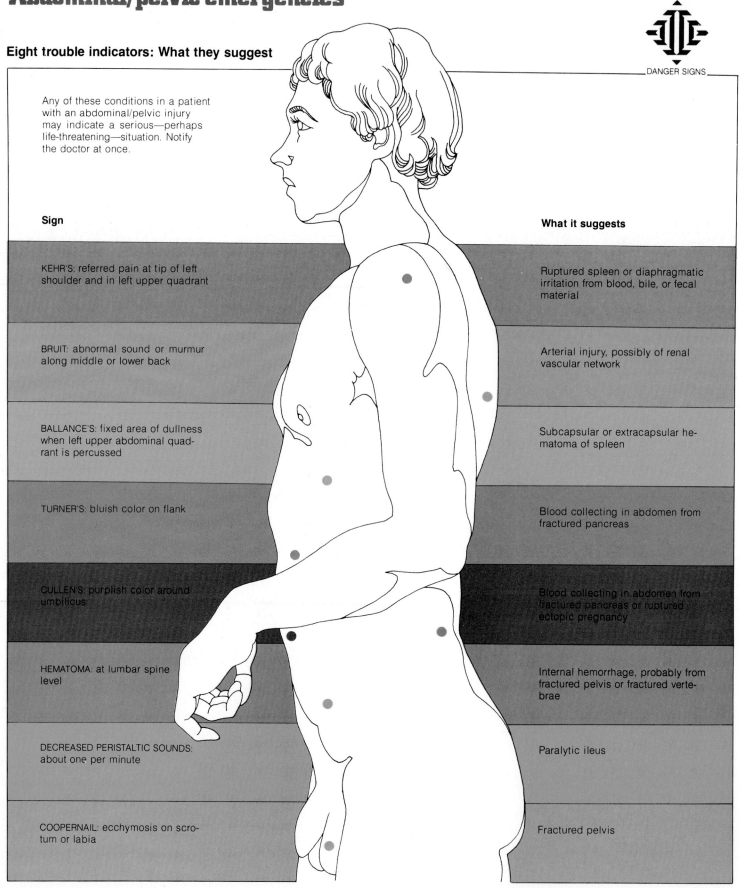

Sign

What it suggests

KEHR'S: referred pain at tip of left shoulder and in left upper quadrant

Ruptured spleen or diaphragmatic irritation from blood, bile, or fecal material

BRUIT: abnormal sound or murmur along middle or lower back

Arterial injury, possibly of renal vascular network

BALLANCE'S: fixed area of dullness when left upper abdominal quadrant is percussed

Subcapsular or extracapsular hematoma of spleen

TURNER'S: bluish color on flank

Blood collecting in abdomen from fractured pancreas

CULLEN'S: purplish color around umbilicus

Blood collecting in abdomen from fractured pancreas or ruptured ectopic pregnancy

HEMATOMA: at lumbar spine level

Internal hemorrhage, probably from fractured pelvis or fractured vertebrae

DECREASED PERISTALTIC SOUNDS: about one per minute

Paralytic ileus

COOPERNAIL: ecchymosis on scrotum or labia

Fractured pelvis

Assisting the doctor with a peritoneal lavage

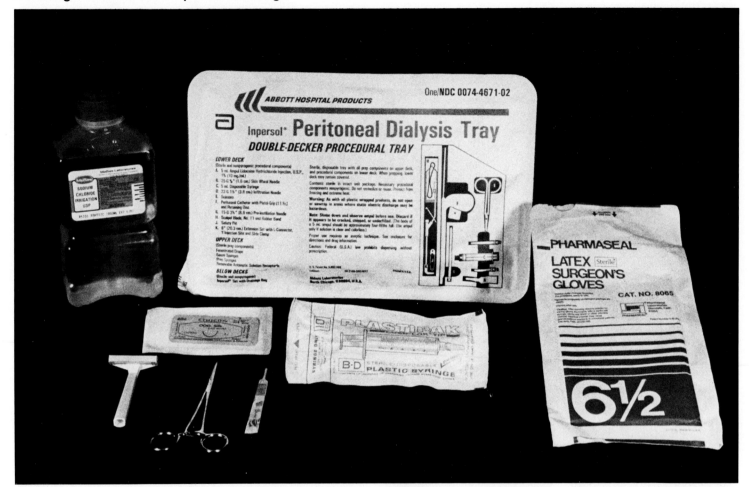

1 *Your patient's condition suggests that he may be bleeding internally in his abdominal/pelvic area. To determine if this is true, the doctor may decide to do a peritoneal lavage. Do you know how to assist him? If you're not sure, read this photostory.*

Important: Don't assume the doctor will order this procedure for every patient with a suspected abdominal hemorrhage. It's contraindicated when a patient may have bowel adhesions from prior surgery.

To prepare for the procedure, gather the necessary equipment: local anesthetic, with 5 cc syringe; 22G and 25G needles; #11 scalpel blade, with handle; a peritoneal dialysis trocar and catheter; a peritoneal dialysis administration set; hemostats; sterile drape, with hole; Betadine solution; razor for prepping the patient's abdomen; 1,000 ml container of the ordered irrigating solution (usually normal saline solution or lactated Ringer's solution); 10 cc syringe; sterile gauze pads in assorted sizes; sterile gloves; silk sutures and suture needle; and a collection bag or bottle (with basin) for drainage.

Nursing tip: If the doctor wants the irrigating solution warmed, place the container in a clean basin filled with water that's approximately 110° F. (45° C.).

Next, explain the procedure to your patient, and reassure him. Make sure he has an empty bladder, to minimize the risk of bladder damage.

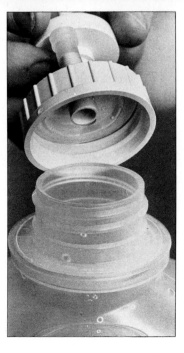

2 Now, using strict aseptic technique, remove the cap from the end of the peritoneal dialysis administration set, and screw it on to the container of irrigating solution.

Important: If you're using an administration set with a Y-connector on the top, make sure the guard on the unused spike stays in place. Also, keep the clamp on that side of the Y-connector closed.

Abdominal/pelvic emergencies

Assisting the doctor with a peritoneal lavage continued

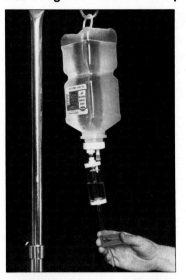

3 Next, hang the container of solution on the I.V. pole, and flush the administration set line to remove any trapped air bubbles. Then, close the main flow clamp until you're ready to attach the line to the catheter. Be sure the clamp is closed on the set's drainage tubing also.

4 Prepare your patient's abdomen. First, shave the area, if necessary. Then, scrub the skin for at least 3 minutes with gauze pads soaked in Betadine solution, as the nurse is doing here.

Exactly which site the doctor will choose to make his incision depends on certain conditions. In most cases, he'll select a site that's midline, just *below* the umbilicus. But if the doctor suspects the patient has an abdominal hematoma in that area—or is pregnant—he'll probably choose a site midline, just *above* the umbilicus.

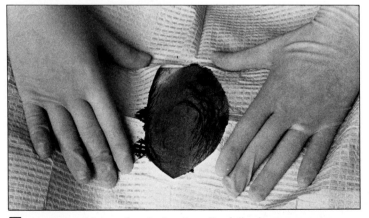

5 Now, stand by as the doctor does the following: covers your patient's abdomen with the sterile drape; anesthetizes the site; makes a small incision in the abdomen, with the scalpel; and then inserts the trocar and catheter.

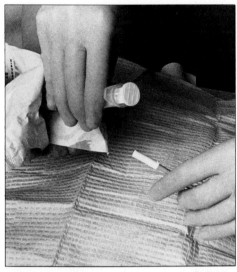

6 Next, hand him the 10 cc syringe so he can draw a fluid sample from the patient's abdomen. Is the fluid bloody? The patient will need immediate surgery. If the fluid isn't bloody, the doctor will continue the peritoneal lavage. Assist by taping the catheter to the patient's abdomen.

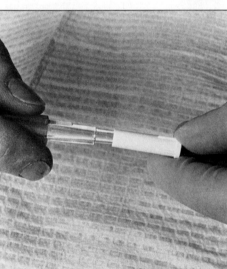

7 When the doctor removes the 10 cc syringe from the catheter, attach the catheter to the primed administration set.

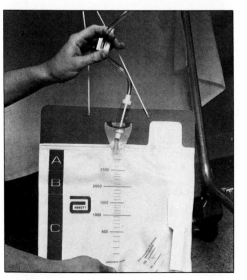

8 Then, clamp the set's drainage tubing, and attach the collection bag to the side of the stretcher, as shown here.

If you're using a collection bottle, place the bottle on the floor, in a clean basin or bucket. Why? If your patient has blood in his abdomen, the drainage will probably overflow the collection bottle.

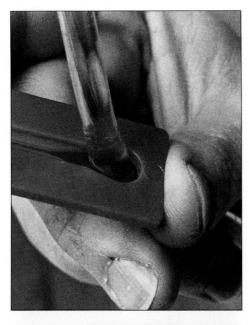

9 Now, open the clamp on the main line of the administration set, and slowly infuse 1,000 ml irrigating solution into the patient's peritoneal cavity. Is your patient a child? Infuse only 10 to 20 ml solution per kg/body weight.

Watch your patient closely. If he complains of abdominal cramps or has sudden diarrhea, stop the infusion immediately. He may have a perforated bowel. Also, stop the infusion if he expresses an urgent need to void. He may have a perforated bladder.

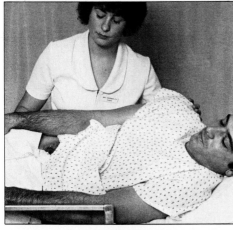

10 When the infusion's completed, close the clamp on the administration set line. Then, gently turn your patient from side to side so the irrigating solution can diffuse through his entire peritoneal cavity.

Important: Never turn a patient who may have a spinal cord injury. Allow him to remain in the same position.

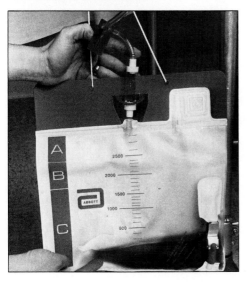

11 After you've turned your patient several times, place him flat on his back again, and open the clamp on the drainage tubing. Carefully check the fluid draining into the collection bag.

Is it bloody? Notify the doctor at once. He'll want you to prepare the patient for immediate surgery.

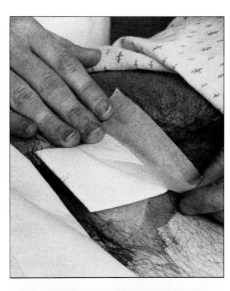

12 When the entire procedure's finished, the doctor will remove the catheter and suture the incision closed.

Apply Betadine ointment to the site, and cover it with a sterile gauze pad. Tape the pad to the patient's abdomen.

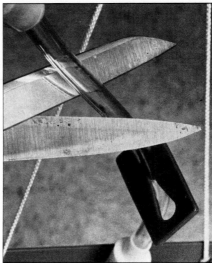

13 The doctor may want to send the entire bag of drainage to the lab for analysis. If he does, prepare it as follows: First, close the clamp on the drainage tubing, and cut the tubing just above the clamp.

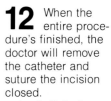

14 Then, label the bag with the patient's name, the date and time, and type of specimen. Attach the appropriate lab slip to the bag, and send it to the lab.

Be sure to document the entire procedure, as well as your patient's reactions to it, in your nurses' notes.

Abdominal/pelvic emergencies

Inserting a Foley catheter

1 *Suppose the doctor orders a Foley catheter for your patient. Do you know how to insert one correctly, using strict aseptic technique? Study the procedure on these pages. (If your patient is a man, check the special considerations on the opposite page before you begin.)*

Assemble the equipment you'll need: a disposable sterile bladder catheter care kit, which includes water-soluble lubricating jelly; plastic-coated drape; drape with precut opening; benzalkonium chloride cleansing solution; gloves; prefilled syringe containing sterile water; and a urine collection bag with drainage tubing attached. Also obtain the correct size Foley catheter.

Before proceeding, reassure your patient, and explain what you're going to do. Wash your hands thoroughly.

4 Slip on the sterile gloves. Then, test the balloon on the Foley catheter by injecting it with sterile water from the prefilled syringe.

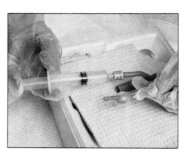

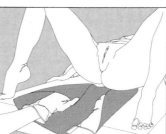

5 Ask the patient to raise her pelvis by pushing down with her feet. Use the technique shown here to place the plastic-coated drape under her buttocks. Take care not to touch the patient's buttocks when you withdraw your hands. Instruct your patient to lower her pelvis onto the drape.

6 Next, position the precut drape so the opening's over the patient's perineal area.

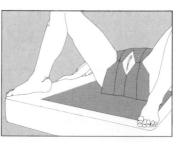

7 Open the packet of lubricating jelly. Squeeze a small amount of jelly onto a sterile gauze pad or into one of the container dividers. Lubricate the first 3" (7.6 cm) of the catheter.

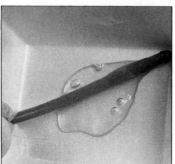

8 Open the cleansing solution packet, and pour the solution over the cotton balls.

2 If your patient's a woman, position her flat on her back, if possible, with her legs bent and her hips adducted. Place her feet 24" (61 cm) apart. Make sure you have strong, direct lighting. Obtain a gooseneck lamp, if necessary.

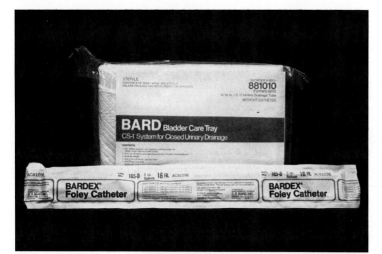

3 Place the sterile catheter kit between her legs, and aseptically open the kit. Now, open the Foley catheter package, and drop the Foley catheter into the open kit.

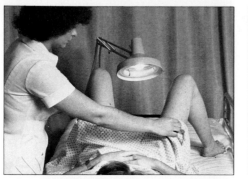

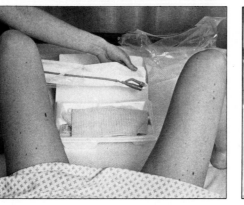

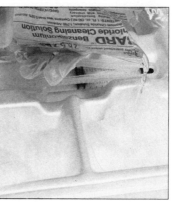

9 If you're right-handed, use your gloved left hand to spread the patient's labia apart. This will expose her urethral meatus. But remember, you must now consider this hand contaminated. Don't touch anything sterile with it.

Be extremely careful not to confuse the patient's urethral opening with her vagina.

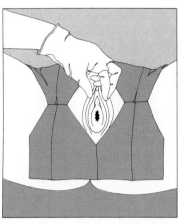

10 With your right hand, use the forceps to pick up a saturated cotton ball. With a downward motion, clean the patient's urethral meatus, as the nurse is doing here. Discard the cotton ball. Now, use another cotton ball to clean around the meatus in an outward, circular motion. Discard this cotton ball, and repeat the procedure, using the remaining cotton balls.

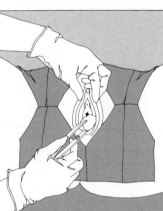

11 Now, grasp the Foley catheter with your uncontaminated hand, and gently insert 2" to 3" (5 to 7.6 cm) into the patient's urethral opening. Never force it. Instead, get a smaller catheter. *Important:* If you must break aseptic technique to do this, start over with a new, sterile kit.

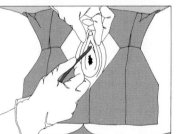

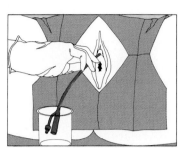

12 As the catheter enters the patient's bladder, release the labia, and place the other end of the catheter in the specimen container. Collect a urine specimen. Take care to grasp the catheter end high enough, so you don't contaminate the specimen.

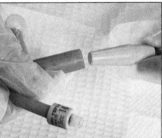

13 Now, connect the open end of the catheter to the drainage tubing and collection bag. Attach the bag to the bed. If more than 1,000 ml urine drains into the bag, clamp the catheter and wait 15 minutes. Allowing any more urine to drain may cause the patient to go into shock.

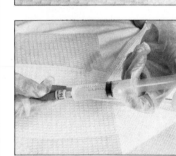

14 Attach the prefilled syringe to the Y portion of the catheter end. Then, inflate the catheter balloon by instilling sterile water into the catheter. (The correct amount of water to instill is printed on the catheter.)

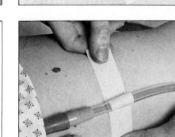

15 Now, secure the catheter. To do this properly, tape the drainage tubing *(not the catheter)* to the patient's inner thigh. If necessary, shave the area, and apply tincture of benzoin first.

Document the procedure in your notes. Start an intake/output record. Send the labeled urine specimen to the lab.

SPECIAL CONSIDERATIONS

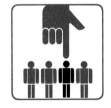

When a man requires catheterization

Some hospitals do not permit a female nurse to catheterize a male patient. But in an emergency, you may have to do it. Follow the same procedure and aseptic technique guidelines as you did for your female patient, with the following modifications:

• Position your patient flat in bed, if possible. Place the plastic-coated drape across the patient's thighs. Now, take the precut drape and pull his penis through the opening. (Consider this hand contaminated.)

• When you clean the area and begin insertion, hold the penis shaft so it's perpendicular to his body. If your patient isn't circumcised, remember to pull back the foreskin before cleansing and insertion. You'll pull it forward again after insertion is complete.

• Lubricate the first 7" to 10" (17.8 to 25.4 cm) of the catheter rather than 3" (7.6 cm), because the male urethra is longer.

• Using the sterile forceps or your sterile hand, advance the catheter along the anterior wall of your patient's urethra. If you note any resistance, increase traction on the penis slightly and try again. Notify the doctor if you continue to have difficulty.

• Advance the catheter 7" to 10" (17.8 to 25.4 cm). If you feel some resistance where the patient's prostate is located, try decreasing the angle of the penis. As soon as urine flows from the catheter, advance the catheter 1" (2.5 cm) more, inflate the balloon, and tape the tubing to the patient's abdomen. Document the procedure, as before. Be sure to send the urine specimen to the laboratory.

Abdominal/pelvic emergencies

How to irrigate a patient's bladder

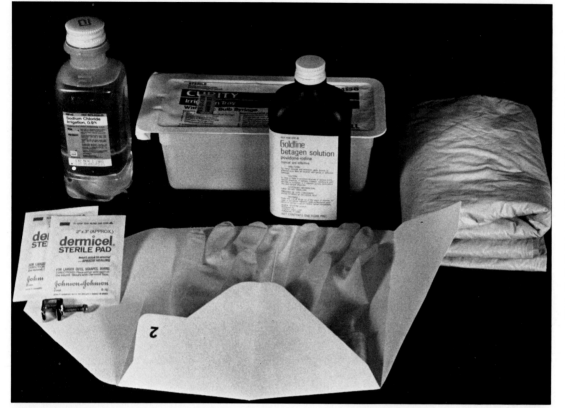

1 *You're working the day shift when 30-year-old Wilma Thatcher arrives in the ED after a car accident. She complains of severe lower back pain and a strong urge to void. But when she does, her urine's scant and bloody. You suspect she may have renal damage. What do you do?*

Notify the doctor immediately. He'll probably want you to insert a Foley catheter. (For details, see page 86). If he also wants you to perform a bladder irrigation, proceed as follows:

First, assemble the equipment you'll need: a sterile irrigation set, the ordered irrigation solution (usually normal saline solution), Betadine solution, sterile gauze pads, bedsaver pad, Hoffman clamp, and sterile gloves.

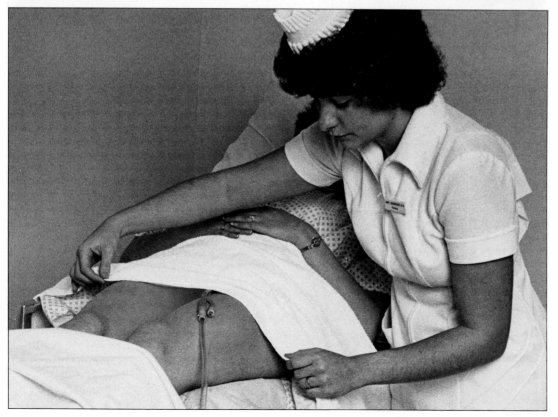

2 Now, explain the procedure and its purpose to your patient. Then, place her in a semi-Fowler's position, and tuck the bedsaver pad under her buttocks and upper thighs.

☛ *Nursing tip:* To avoid exposing her unnecessarily, drape a towel or sheet over her pubic area, as shown here.

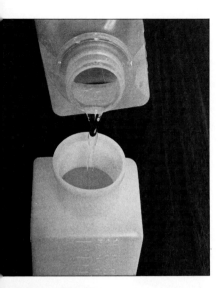

3 Next, wash your hands thoroughly. Unwrap the equipment, using aseptic technique. Then, open the bottle of normal saline solution, and pour 500 ml into the solution container. Take care not to touch the inside of the container with the bottle. Doing so may contaminate it.

Check the solution's temperature to make sure it's no warmer than body temperature.

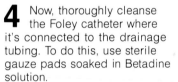

4 Now, thoroughly cleanse the Foley catheter where it's connected to the drainage tubing. To do this, use sterile gauze pads soaked in Betadine solution.

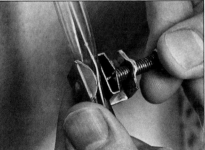

5 Next, clamp the drainage tubing closed with a Hoffman clamp, as shown here. Carefully disconnect the tubing from the Foley catheter. Then, holding the catheter upright to keep it sterile, cap the tubing with a sterile rubber tip.

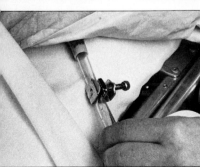

6 Tuck the capped tubing under the bedsaver pad to keep it from touching the floor. Remember, you must perform the entire procedure using aseptic technique.

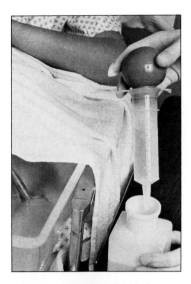

7 Now, position the sterile drainage basin under the Foley catheter, and make sure it's secure. Put on the sterile gloves, and draw about 50 ml of irrigating solution into the bulb syringe.

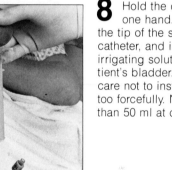

8 Hold the catheter steady in one hand. Then, insert the tip of the syringe into the catheter, and instill 50 ml of irrigating solution into your patient's bladder. *Important:* Take care not to instill the solution too forcefully. Never instill more than 50 ml at one time.

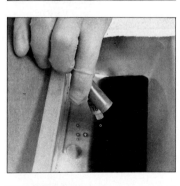

9 Now, remove the syringe, and position the end of the catheter over the drainage basin. Collect the irrigation return in the basin, and note its appearance. Then, repeat the irrigation procedure until the returning fluid is clear.

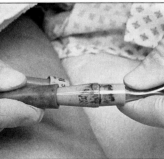

10 Finally, clean the Foley catheter with Betadine-soaked gauze pads, and reconnect the drainage tubing. Document the type and amount of irrigation solution used; the color of the returning fluid; the number of blood clots, if any; and the patient's reaction to the procedure.

Arm and leg emergencies

Do you know how to give emergency care to a patient with an injured arm or leg? For example, suppose he arrives in the ED with a partially—or completely—severed hand. Do you know what to do first? How do you prepare him for surgery? What about replantation? How do you care for the amputated hand?

And what about other injuries? How do you apply Buck's extension to a patient with a dislocated hip? Can you recognize a comminuted fracture? How do you check the pressure in an air splint? If you're not sure, you need to read the following pages. In them, you'll find the answers to all these important questions ... plus much, much more.

MINI-ASSESSMENT

Does your patient have a bone fracture?

Assessing a patient's injuries? You'll know for certain he has a bone fracture if a bone's protruding from his skin. But in many cases, a bone fracture is less obvious. So, teach yourself to *suspect* a possible bone fracture if your patient has any of the following signs or symptoms in an injured arm or leg:
• obvious deformity from injury; for example, angulation, rotation, shortening
• swelling or pain (especially on movement)
• decreased sensations
• partial or complete loss of motor function
• skin coolness or blanching.

If you notice any of the above, notify the doctor immediately. He'll want the patient to have an X-ray to confirm the fracture's presence and type.

How can you help in the meantime? Reassure your patient, and explain what you're going to do. Then, apply a splint to his injured limb *before* he's taken to X-ray. (For complete instructions on how to pad and apply a splint, see page 94 and 95.)

Suppose the bone is protruding from the patient's skin. *Before you apply the splint,* control the bleeding and cover the open wound with a sterile dressing. Take care to use aseptic technique.

For all cases, check your patient's vital signs periodically. Document your findings, including information about the accident, in your nurses' notes.

For more information about the types of fractures patients may have, see the chart on these pages.

Nurses' guide to fractures

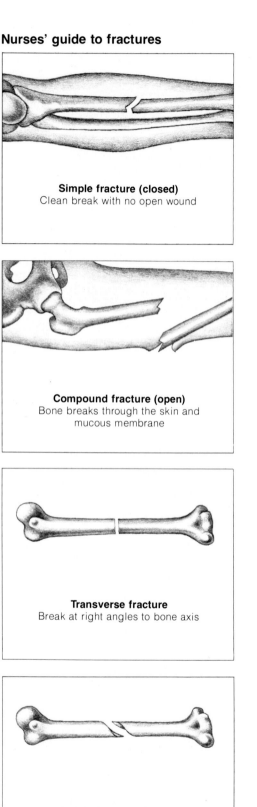

Simple fracture (closed)
Clean break with no open wound

Compound fracture (open)
Bone breaks through the skin and mucous membrane

Transverse fracture
Break at right angles to bone axis

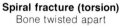

Spiral fracture (torsion)
Bone twisted apart

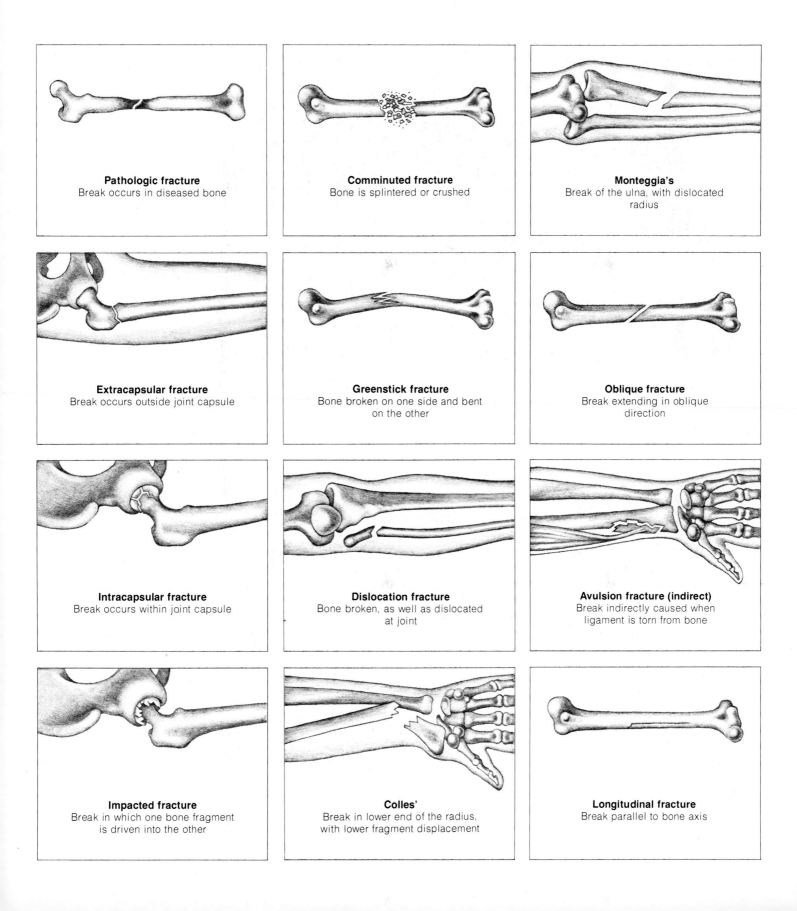

Pathologic fracture
Break occurs in diseased bone

Comminuted fracture
Bone is splintered or crushed

Monteggia's
Break of the ulna, with dislocated radius

Extracapsular fracture
Break occurs outside joint capsule

Greenstick fracture
Bone broken on one side and bent on the other

Oblique fracture
Break extending in oblique direction

Intracapsular fracture
Break occurs within joint capsule

Dislocation fracture
Bone broken, as well as dislocated at joint

Avulsion fracture (indirect)
Break indirectly caused when ligament is torn from bone

Impacted fracture
Break in which one bone fragment is driven into the other

Colles'
Break in lower end of the radius, with lower fragment displacement

Longitudinal fracture
Break parallel to bone axis

Arm and leg emergencies

Immobilizing an injured extremity

To properly immobilize an injured extremity requires know-how and practice. Depending on the patient's injury, you may have to apply a sling, splint, swathe, or traction device. Are you uncertain about the procedure used for each? Don't be. Read the following photo-stories to learn what's required.

Remember, however, to check your patient before applying any of these devices. Remove any tight clothing or jewelry she may be wearing, and cover any open wounds with sterile dressings.

How to apply a sling

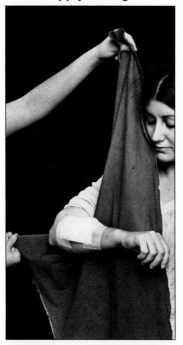

1 *If your patient has an injured shoulder or arm, use a sling to immobilize it.* To properly apply a sling, position the triangle's longest side along your patient's midline. Place the triangle's point at her elbow, as shown here. Then, cradle her injured arm between the two ends.

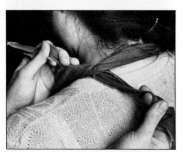

2 Now, knot the other two ends of the sling loosely but securely around your patient's neck. Use a safety pin to fasten the sling at her elbow.

☎ *Nursing tip:* Never position the knot in the center back of your patient's neck, as you may cause nerve damage.

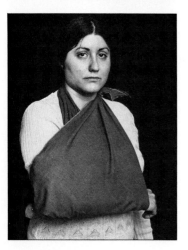

3 When the sling's applied properly, the patient's injured arm should be immobilized at a 90° angle, as shown here. Encourage your patient to maintain muscle tone in her injured arm. One way she can do this is by squeezing a tennis ball.

How to apply a swathe

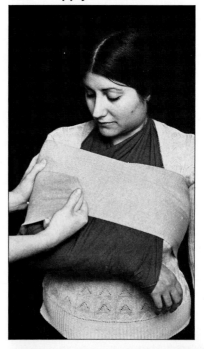

1 *To immobilize an injured shoulder or provide additional support for an arm that's already in a sling, apply a swathe.* To do this, position the patient's injured arm or shoulder as close as possible to her body. Then, wrap a wide elastic bandage several times *over* her arm and *around* her upper torso, as shown here. However, take care not to cover her *uninjured* arm, or her hand and wrist.

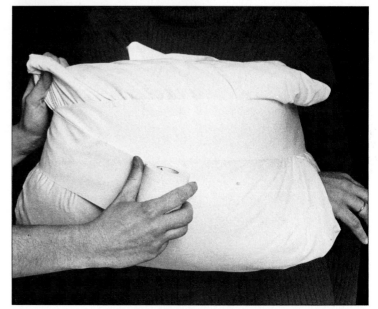

2 Suppose you don't have a sling or a swathe handy. Immobilize an injured arm or shoulder with a pillow and adhesive tape. To do this, cradle your patient's arm lengthwise on the pillow. Then, bring the pillow's sides together, and wrap with adhesive tape. Secure the sling to your patient's body with more tape, as shown in this photo.

How to apply a figure-eight strap

1 *Does your patient have a clavicle fracture or shoulder injury? If so, use a figure-eight strap to immobilize it.* You can use a commercially made figure-eight strap, or make your own. To use the commercially made strap, wrap the strap ends over your patient's shoulder and under her arms. Then, fasten the Velcro ends in the back, as shown here.

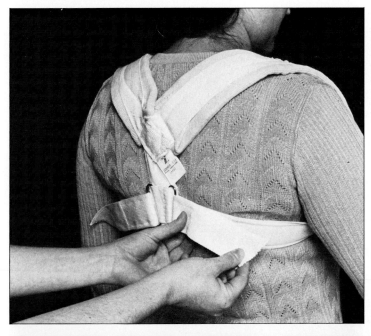

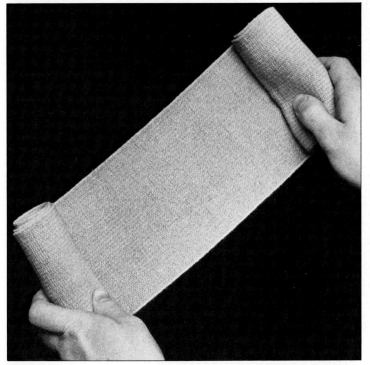

2 To make your own figure-eight strap, you'll need a 4' (120 cm) length of elastic bandage or stockinette (less if your patient's a child). Then carefully roll both ends to the center of the bandage.

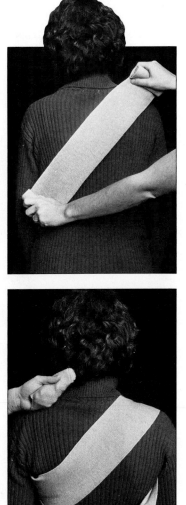

3 Now, place the center of the bandage at the center of your patient's back. Bring the left end of the bandage under her left arm and the right end over her right shoulder.

4 Next, bring the left end of the bandage up and over the patient's left shoulder, toward her back. At the same time, bring the right end under the patient's right arm, toward her back.

5 Bring both ends to your patient's center back. Fasten the straps together with safety pins.
Important: Make sure the strap is wrapped tightly enough to ensure proper shoulder alignment. However, don't wrap so tightly that you constrict your patient's circulation.

Arm and leg emergencies

How to apply an air splint

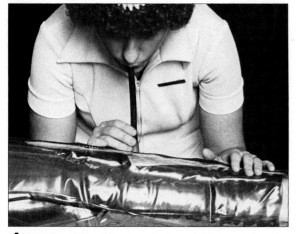

1 *Here's still another way to immobilize an injured arm or leg: use an air splint.* Slip the deflated splint on the patient's injured limb, and zip it closed. Now, inflate the splint by blowing air into the nozzle.

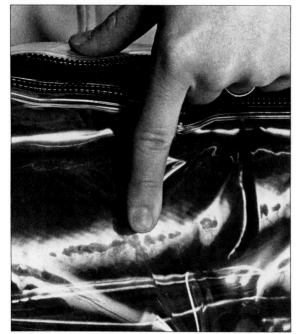

2 When it's inflated, check the air pressure. To do this, depress the inflated splint with your fingertips. If you can indent the plastic approximately ½″ (1.3 cm), the splint's properly inflated.

To further guard against constriction caused by an overinflated air splint, check the skin color and temperature of your patient's toes every 15 minutes. If you suspect a problem, slowly release some air from the splint, until the pressure's correct. Periodically, recheck it, using the method described above.

📨 *Nursing tip:* Never apply any splint without first padding the patient's joints with towels or gauze. Careful padding will minimize the risk of skin breakdown.

How to apply a preformed splint

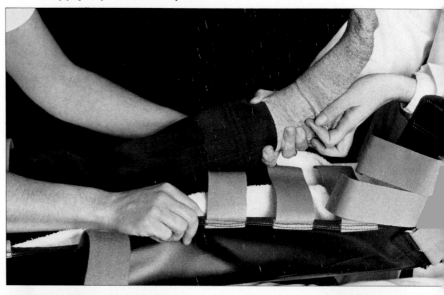

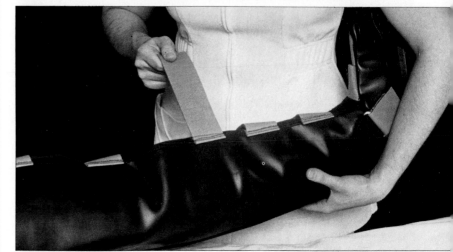

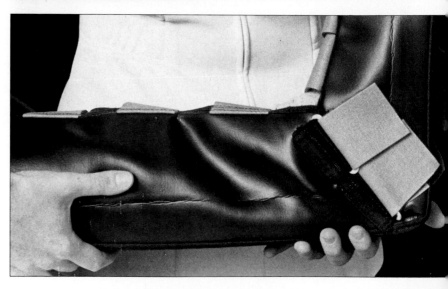

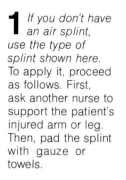

How to improvise a splint

1 *If you don't have an air splint, use the type of splint shown here.* To apply it, proceed as follows. First, ask another nurse to support the patient's injured arm or leg. Then, pad the splint with gauze or towels.

2 Place the splint under the injured limb. Secure the splint with Velcro bandages or straps, as the nurse is doing here.

3 Gently attempt to move the splinted limb into a functional anatomical position. However, *don't force it.* Never try to straighten an injured arm or leg that's severely angulated. If you do, you may cause further damage.

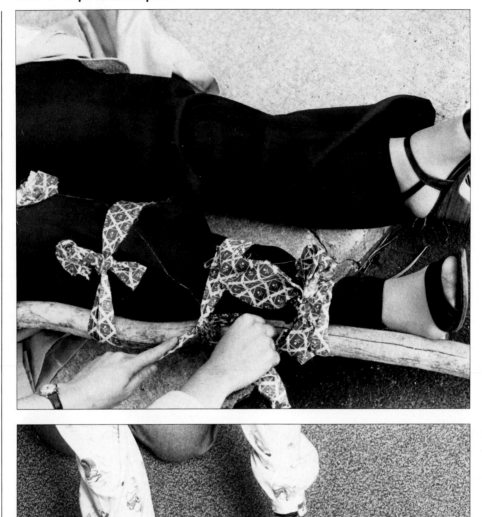

1 *If you're outside the hospital when such an emergency occurs, you may have to improvise a splint.*
To do so, use rolled up newspapers, a tree limb, or a mop handle. Pad the splint with clothing. Then, secure the improvised splint to the patient's injured arm or leg with tape or cloth strips. *Never use rope or twine, because these may constrict her circulation.*

2 Suppose you don't have a newspaper, tree limb, or mop handle. Here's another improvisation you can use if your patient has an injured leg: Temporarily splint it by wrapping it against her *uninjured* leg.

Arm and leg emergencies

Applying traction with Buck's extension

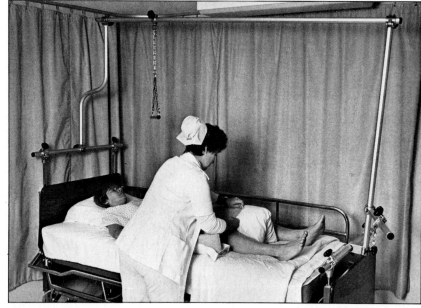

1 *Does your patient have a dislocated hip? If so, the doctor may order a Buck's extension to immobilize it. Do you know how to apply it? This step-by-step photostory will tell you:*

First, following manufacturer's instructions, assemble and attach the traction apparatus to the bed. Position your patient flat on her back, making sure her body is properly supported and aligned. Remove any temporary splinting devices, as the nurse is doing here.

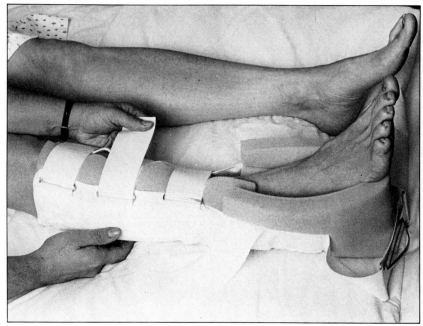

2 Now, gently place your patient's injured leg in the traction's open splint. *Important:* Most splints of this type are already padded with foam rubber. If the one you're using isn't, add padding before you begin.

Next, secure the splint with the fasteners, as shown here.

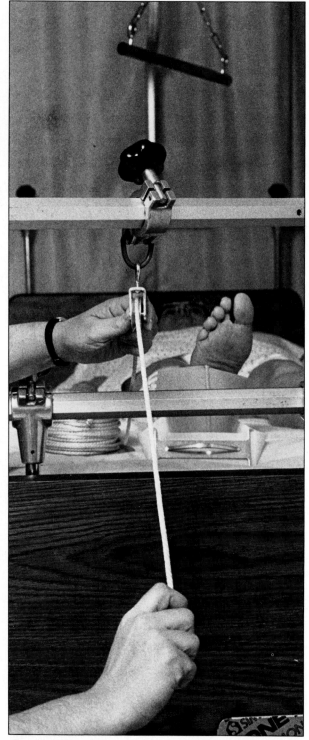

3 With the piece of rope, measure the distance from your patient's foot, to about 12" (30.5 cm) over the pulley. Then, cut the rope to the desired length.

⊜ *Nursing tip:* To keep the rope from fraying, knot each end.

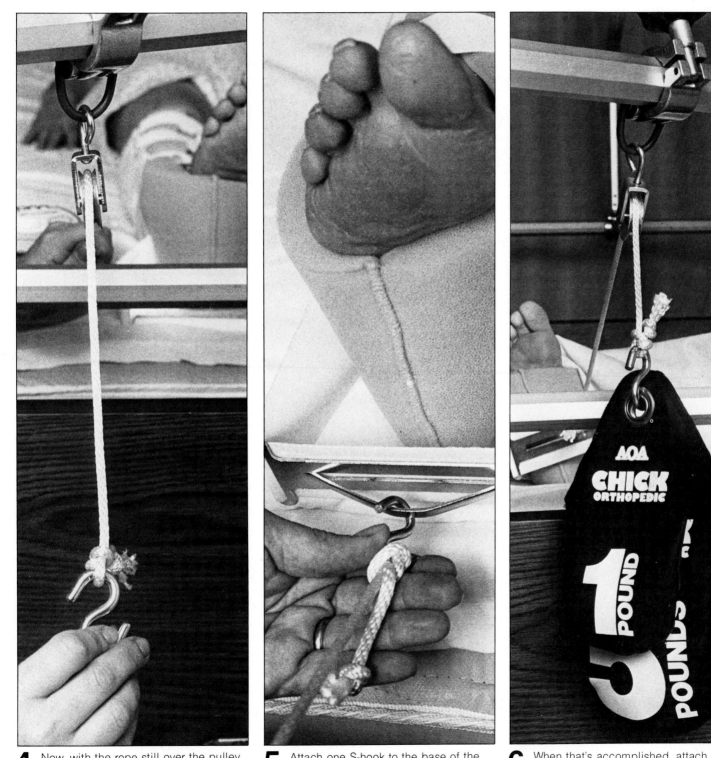

4 Now, with the rope still over the pulley, carefully form a slipknot at each end. Place an S-hook in each slipknot, and make sure it's secure.

5 Attach one S-hook to the base of the splint, as shown here. Make sure the top part of the hook is pointing up, to keep it from slipping off the splint.

6 When that's accomplished, attach the prescribed amount of weight to the rope that's over the pulley. Release the weights carefully. Be sure they hang freely, as shown in this photo. *Important:* Never let the weights touch the floor.

Arm and leg emergencies

Splinting an injured hip

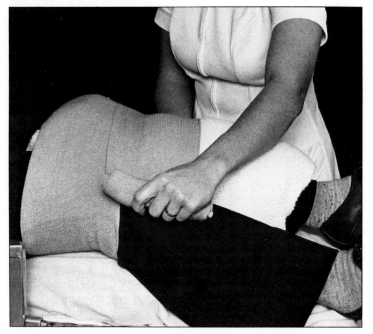

If you suspect your patient has a fractured or dislocated hip, you may have to improvise a hip splint until medical help's available.

To do this, position a pillow or folded blanket between your patient's legs. Then, wrap elastic bandages or cravats around both legs, as shown here.

Do's and don'ts of fracture care

• Do ease your patient's pain and distress by explaining what you're going to do.
• Don't straighten a severely angulated extremity before immobilizing it.
• Don't push protruding bone ends into your patient's skin when you immobilize the injured extremity.
• Do remember to pad the splint before you apply it.
• Don't constrict your patient's circulation when you immobilize his injured part.
• Do check your patient's immobilized extremity every 15 minutes for possible temperature and color changes.
• Do elevate the patient's injured extremity above his heart after you splint it, to decrease risk of edema.
• Do look for signs that your patient may have internal hemorrhaging, increased pain, or shock. For example, stay alert for personality changes, restlessness, or irritability.
• Do give your patient medication for pain, as ordered by the doctor.
• Do notify the doctor if you have problems with your patient's traction device.

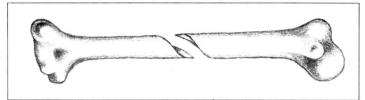

Treating a soft-tissue injury

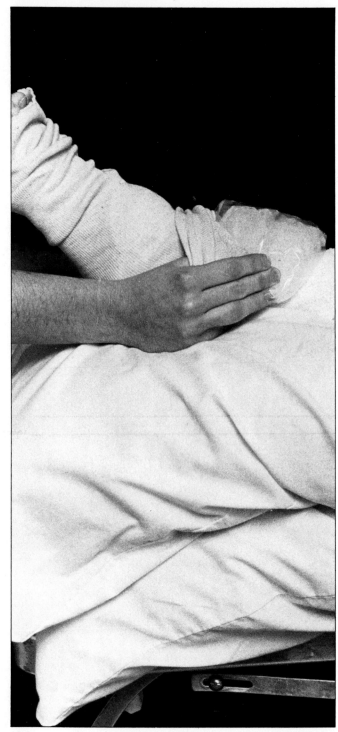

1 *Do you know how to care for a patient with a sprained ankle or other soft-tissue injury? Here's what to do:*
First, wrap a dry towel around your patient's injured extremity. (In this case, let's assume it's a sprained ankle.) Then, elevate it above her heart level. Apply an ice bag or cold compress to the area to combat swelling and pain. Pull a stockinette over the bag.

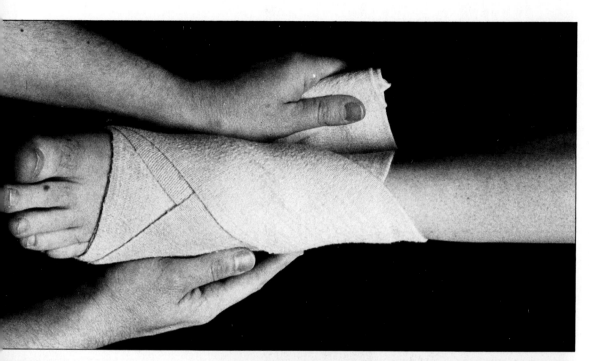

2 Now, the doctor may order an X-ray, to see if the bone has been fractured. Depending on what the X-ray shows, he may instruct you to wrap the ankle.

To do this, remove ice packs. Wrap an elastic bandage around your patient's ankle in a figure-eight style, keeping her heel and toes exposed. Note: Some doctors prefer that the heel be included in the wrap. Remember, your patient will probably have to remove and reapply the elastic bandage at home. So, as you wrap her ankle, explain what you're doing.

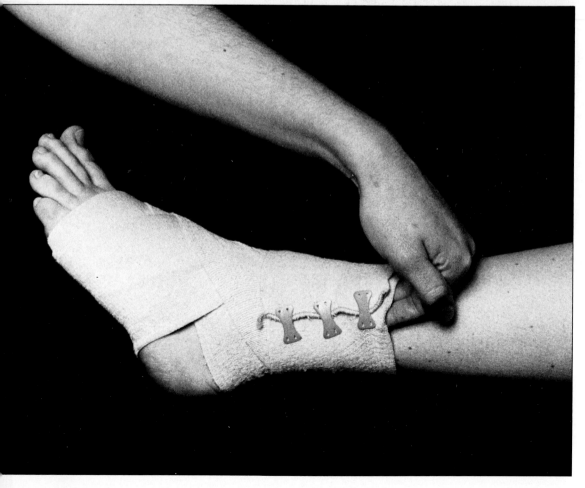

3 Tell your patient not to wrap too tightly. As a check for tightness, show her how to slip her fingers between the bandage and her ankle.

When the ankle's wrapped, reapply the ice bag, and pull the stockinette over the bag. Instruct your patient to apply ice intermittently over the next 12 to 36 hours.

Ⓢ *Nursing tip:* Use Ziploc® bags for ice, so the patient can take the ice home with her. Document the procedure in your nurses' notes, including information about how the accident occurred.

Another important reminder: Instruct your patient to avoid putting weight on her affected ankle for a few days, as this may increase tissue damage.

Patient teaching

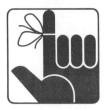

How to use crutches
Dear Patient:
Has the doctor given you crutches? If used properly, these crutches will help you reduce or eliminate the amount of weight you put on your injured leg or foot.

But first, find out if the crutches are right for you. Check them out by following these guidelines:
• Make sure the crutches are ready to use. You'll need rubber suction cups placed over the wooden crutch tips to prevent sliding. You'll also need rubber pads on the underarm pieces, to make them more comfortable. You may also ask the nurse to pad the hand supports.
• Are the crutches the right size? When you're standing—with the crutch tips 6" (15.2 cm) from the sides of your feet—underarm pieces should be about 1" to 1½" (two finger-widths or 2.5 to 3.8 cm) *below* your armpits. If they touch your armpits, ask the nurse to adjust the length.
• Check the placement of the hand supports. When you grasp them, your arms should be slightly bent—*never* straight. When you're certain the crutches are the right size and properly padded, let the nurse show you how to use them. But remember, crutch-walking requires practice. Don't get discouraged if you have difficulty at first.

Here are some hints to help you get started:
• Always use your *arms* to support your weight, not the top part of the crutch. If you feel any tingling or numbness in your upper torso, you're probably using the crutches incorrectly. Or they may be the wrong size.
• Before you attempt walking with your crutches, lean your body slightly forward.
• Always keep the crutches in front of you. Doing so will ensure better balance. Now, study the instructions with the illustrations on these pages to find out how to use your crutches.

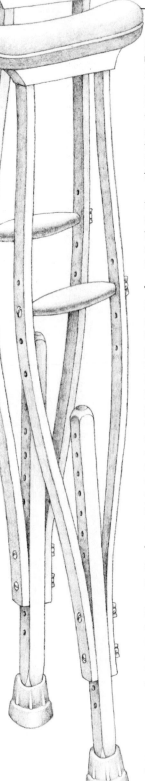

How to crutch-walk using the three-point gait
If the doctor says you can put some weight on your injured leg, he'll probably want you to crutch-walk with a three-point gait. Read the captions with these illustrations to discover how to do this.

Note: Depending on the type of injury you have, the doctor may also want you to learn a two-point and a four-point gait. (Ask the nurse about these.)

How to use your crutches on stairs
Sooner or later, you'll have to get up and down stairs, using your crutches. Assuming the bannister is on the right, here's how to proceed:
• First, stand at the bottom of the stairs, and shift your crutches to your left hand.
• Grasp the bannister firmly with your right hand. Using your left hand, carefully support your weight on the crutches.

Getting in and out of a chair
If you're on crutches, you'll need practice getting in and out of a chair. Before you begin, study the illustrations at the right. Then, follow these guidelines:
• Select the chair carefully. Make sure it's sturdy and has arms. Never attempt to sit in a chair that's on casters.
• Now, stand with your back toward the chair. Slowly move backward until you feel

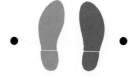 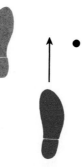 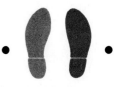

With the crutches in place, stand straight, with your shoulders relaxed and your arms slightly bent. Use your hands to support your weight.

Now, swing your injured leg in front of you at the same time you move the crutches forward. Maintain your balance by placing some weight on your uninjured leg.

Balance your weight on both crutches as you swing your uninjured leg forward.

Advance your uninjured leg to the position shown here. Put your weight on this leg as you bring your crutches forward.

Then, advance your injured leg to the first position, and repeat the procedure.

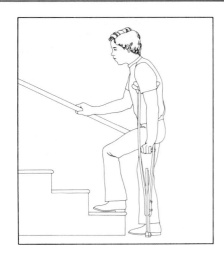 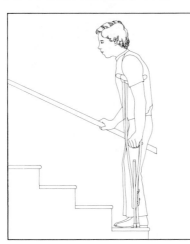

- Now, hop up onto the first step with your uninjured leg. (Your injured leg will move up at the same time.)
- Support your weight on that leg as you grasp the bannister tightly.
- Swing your crutches up onto the first step (see second illustration).
- Now, hop up onto the second step with your uninjured leg.
- Continue the procedure as before, but go slowly to avoid losing your balance.

To get down the stairs, reverse the guidelines you've just learned. But, when you do, remember that you *always advance the crutches and your injured leg first*.

the back of your knees touch the front edge of the chair.
- Now, transfer both crutches to the hand that's next to your *injured* leg.
- As you support your weight on the crutches, reach back with your other hand, and grasp the chair arm. Lower yourself into the chair slowly.
- To get up from the chair, bring both crutches alongside your injured leg. With the hand on this side, grasp the hand supports of the crutches firmly. Place your other hand on the arm of the chair, and push yourself up.
- Once you're upright, transfer one of the crutches to your uninjured side, and get ready to walk.

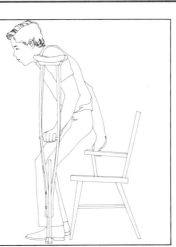 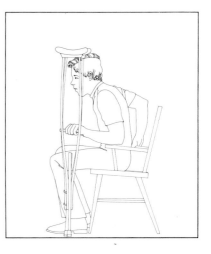

Gastric intubation and lavage

What is a nontraumatic emergency? A sudden physiologic change in the patient's condition that's *not* caused by physical injury. Like other emergencies, it requires immediate treatment.

What's *your* special challenge in a nontraumatic emergency? Recognizing and caring for the patient's problem quickly and effectively. And that's not easy, because in most cases, you won't be able to see what's wrong.

To help you, we've included the information on these pages. In the following photostories and charts, you'll find out how to identify and cope with such nontraumatic emergencies as hypoglycemia, anaphylactic shock, and pulmonary edema. And, you'll learn about many of the necessary procedures required; for example, how to insert a nasogastric tube, how to perform a gastric lavage, and how to apply rotating tourniquets.

How to insert a nasogastric tube

1 *Your patient may need a nasogastric tube inserted for almost any nontraumatic emergency. If the doctor orders such a tube, will you know how to insert it? This photostory will show you what to do.*

Begin by washing your hands thoroughly. Remember, although this is not a sterile procedure, you should make every effort to prevent contamination. Now, gather the equipment shown in this photo: French size 12 to 18 nasogastric tube or Salem sump tube, penlight, basin with ice, Hoffman clamps, cup of water with straw, bulb syringe, towel, water-soluble lubricating jelly, gauze pads, nonallergenic tape, small rubber band, and safety pin. (If your patient's a child, you'll need a smaller size tube.)

Test the tube's patency by running water through it. Then, examine it closely for roughness or ragged edges.

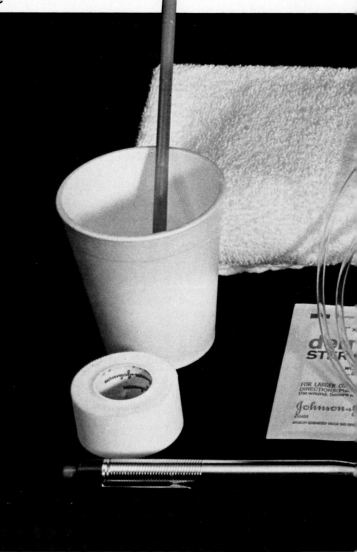

2 Is the nasogastric tube you've selected made of one of the newer plastics? It may be too stiff to insert gently. If it is, place it in warm water for several minutes. On the other hand, if the tube seems too pliant, chill it in a basin of ice, as shown here.

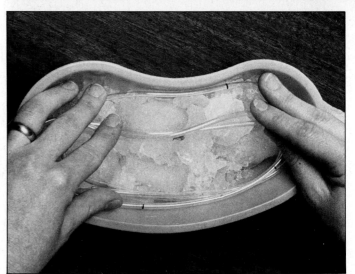

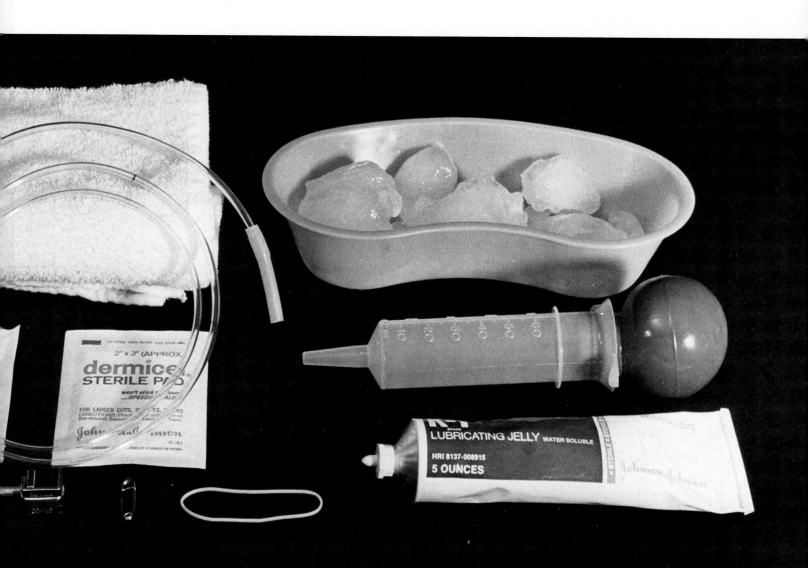

3 Tell your patient what you're going to do in words she can understand. Encourage her questions and answer them honestly. Warn her that the procedure will be uncomfortable, and agree on a signal she can use if she wants you to stop for a moment.

Seat your patient in a high Fowler's position, with her neck hyperextended, as shown here. Use bedsaver pads or a towel to protect her gown and the bed linen. Give her a handful of tissues, because this procedure may cause tearing. Also make sure she has an emesis basin handy, in case she vomits.

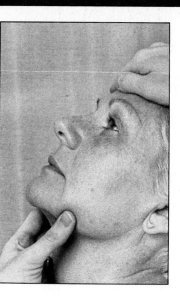

4 Now, use a penlight to check your patient's nostrils. Look for any deformities or obstructions that may make it difficult or impossible to insert the nasogastric tube. If neither nostril is patent, notify the doctor. But if all seems well, proceed to the next step.

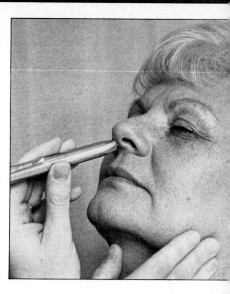

Gastric intubation and lavage

How to insert a nasogastric tube continued

5 Use a two-step method to determine how much tube to insert. To do this, first use the tube to measure the distance from the patient's earlobe to the tip of her nose, as shown here. Then, measure the distance from her earlobe to the bottom of her xiphoid process. Total these two measurements, and mark the correct length on the tube with adhesive tape.

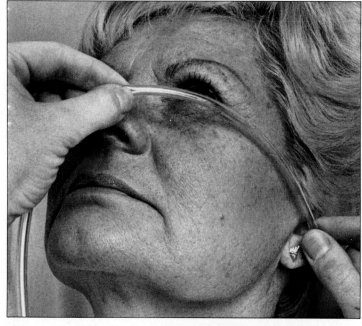

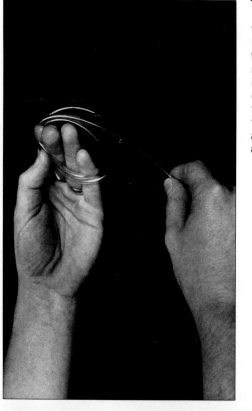

7 Hold the tube 6" (15.2 cm) from its tip. Roll it between your fingers to discover its natural curve. If none is present, shape a curve yourself by tightly coiling the first 5" (12.7 cm) around your fingers, as shown here.

6 If your patient's a child, measure the distance from the tip of his nose to his earlobe, then from his earlobe to a point midway between his xiphoid process and his umbilicus. Total these measurements as before.

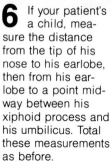

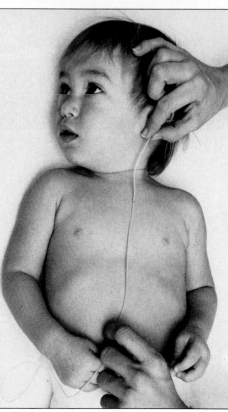

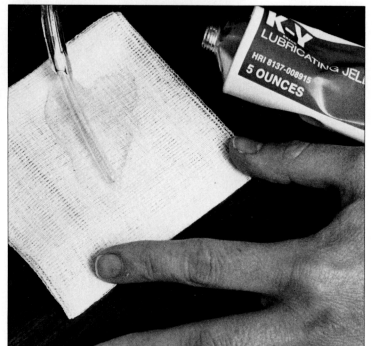

8 Now, generously lubricate the first 6" (15.2 cm) of the tube with water-soluble jelly. *Important:* Never lubricate a nasogastric tube with mineral oil. The patient could aspirate the oil and develop respiratory complications.

9 Now you're ready to insert the tube. Tell your patient to hold her head still. Then, insert the tube into one of her nostrils, and gently advance it toward the posterior nasopharynx. You'll find this easier if you direct the tube toward the patient's ear, not toward her other nostril.

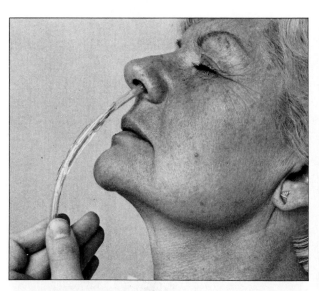

10 As you feel the tube approach the nasopharyngeal junction, rotate it 180° inward, toward the other nostril. Continue to advance it gently until it's in the nasopharynx, pointing toward the esophagus. Work very slowly so the patient won't vomit. *Important:* If you feel resistance at any point in the nasal passage, stop the procedure at once and withdraw the tube. Relubricate it and try the other nostril (provided it's patent).

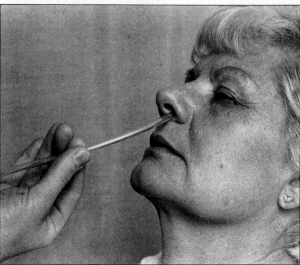

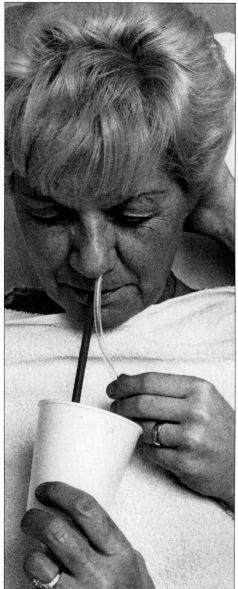

11 Suppose your conscious patient gags during the procedure. To prevent her from vomiting, stop advancing the tube, and tell her to take several deep breaths. Or, ask her to swallow short sips of water through a straw. Both actions will relax the pharynx and calm the gag reflex. The water will also help lubricate the tube. If she continues to gag, look inside her mouth with the penlight. The tube may be coiled in her throat. If it is, withdraw it until it's straight.

Reassure the patient, and let her rest for a few moments before continuing with the procedure.

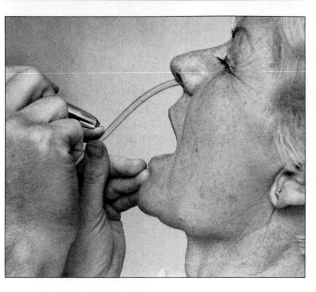

12 Next, ask her to tilt her head forward slightly. This action will close her trachea and open her esophagus. Advance the tube through her oropharynx into her esophagus.

Now, you're ready to advance the tube down the esophagus to the stomach. To make this part of the procedure easier for you and the patient, ask her to sip water or chew ice chips. Then, advance the tubing 3″ to 5″ (7.6 to 12.7 cm) each time she swallows. Of course, if your patient's unconscious, you would never give her any liquids.

🖘 *Nursing tip:* If your patient isn't permitted to drink water, ask her to swallow at a given signal.

Gastric intubation and lavage

How to insert a nasogastric tube continued

13 Continue inserting the tube until you reach the premeasured tape mark.
Important: If you can't insert the tube to the entire measured length, it's probably in the patient's trachea, not her esophagus. Or, it may be curled in the back of her throat. Signs of respiratory distress or vapor in the tubing may also indicate that the tube's in the trachea. Withdraw it at once.

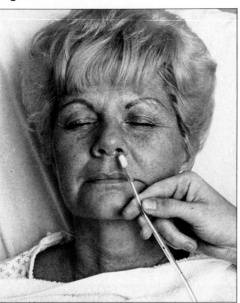

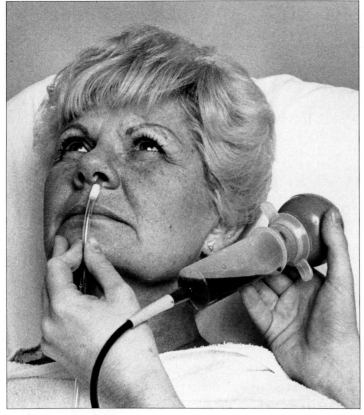

14 Check to make sure the tube's properly placed. To do this, attach a syringe to the end of the tube, and attempt to aspirate gastric fluid. If no fluid can be withdrawn, the tube is probably in the patient's lung. Withdraw it immediately. (For other ways to check proper tube placement, see the opposite page.) Remember to be particularly careful about tube placement in an unconscious patient.

15 When you're sure the tube's in the stomach, secure it as follows: Cut a 1" (2.5 cm) wide strip of nonallergenic tape 3" (7.6 cm) long. Split it lengthwise, leaving a small tab intact at one end (see inset). Then, apply tincture of benzoin to the patient's nose, and wait until it feels tacky. Then, apply the tab end of the tape over the benzoin, as shown here. Crisscross the split ends of the tape under the tube and up onto the patient's nose.
Never tape the tube to the patient's forehead. Doing so can cause a pressure sore in the nasal passage.

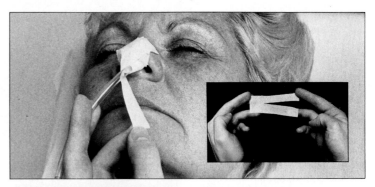

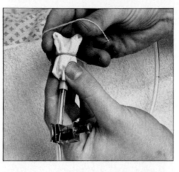

16 Next, clamp or plug the end of the tubing. Then cover it with gauze unless the patient feels nauseated. In that case, leave the end of the tube open and attach to a drainage bag to provide an outlet for vomitus. If you've inserted a Salem sump tube, the doctor will probably want you to attach it to the suctioning machine for intermittent suction.

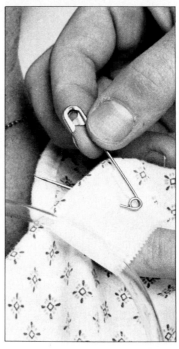

17 Don't permit the tube to dangle and possibly become dislodged. To prevent this, wrap adhesive tape near the end of the tubing, leaving a tab. Then, use a safety pin to pin the tab to the patient's gown, just below her shoulder.
Nursing tip: As an alternate method, loop a rubber band around the tube in slipknot fashion. Pin the rubber band to the patient's gown.
Finally, document the procedure. Then, for the patient's comfort and well-being, provide nose and mouth care. Minimize irritation by placing a small amount of water-soluble lubricating jelly in each nostril. Prevent pressure sores by checking your patient regularly to make sure the tubing's positioned comfortably. Encourage the patient to brush her teeth several times a day.

Checking nasogastric tube placement

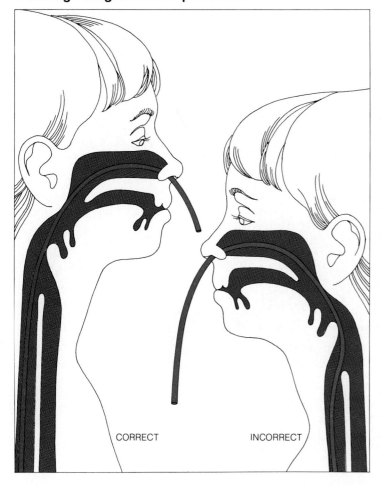

CORRECT   INCORRECT

You've just inserted a nasogastric tube. What's your next step? Make sure the tube's in the patient's stomach and not her lung. Here are some ways you can check. Remember, you'll need to try at least two of these tests to verify correct placement.

Here's the first test, which we already explained in part on the opposite page. To perform it, attach a syringe to the tube, and try to aspirate gastric fluid. If no fluid can be aspirated, withdraw the tube slightly. The end of the tube may be against the stomach wall. Try again. If you still can't aspirate gastric fluid, withdraw the tube completely. It's probably in the patient's lung.

However, don't assume that the tube is properly placed if you *can* aspirate gastric fluid. If your patient has vomited recently, she may have gastric fluid in her lung. Try another test.

Now, consider these other ways to check for correct tube placement:
• Place a stethoscope over the patient's stomach. Attach a syringe to the nasogastric tube, and inject about 15 ml of air. Listen for the sound of air entering the patient's stomach. If you don't hear anything, the tube may be improperly placed in her lung.
• Ask a conscious patient to hum. If she can't, the tube may have entered her trachea and separated her vocal cords.
• Hold the end of the nasogastric tube to your ear. If the tube's in the patient's stomach, you'll hear nothing. If it's in her lung, you'll hear crackling noises.

Some nurses place the end of the tube in a glass of water and watch for air bubbles as the patient exhales. But we don't recommend this method, because we consider it unreliable and dangerous. If the tube is incorrectly placed in the patient's lung, she could aspirate water when she inhales.

As we said earlier, try at least two of these tests to confirm correct placement before you proceed further—or before you administer anything through the tube. If the test results suggest that the tube's in the patient's lung, withdraw it immediately and try again.

Performing a gastric lavage

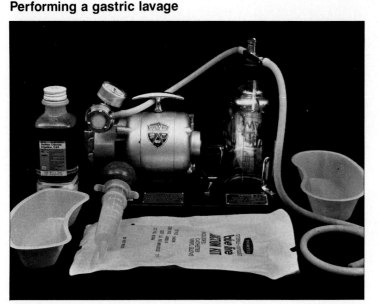

1 *A man who's accidentally overdosed himself with medication has just been admitted to the emergency department where you work. How can you help him?* First, insert a nasogastric tube, using the procedure we've just outlined. Then, get ready to perform a gastric lavage, if the doctor orders one.

Caution: Never perform a gastric lavage on a patient who's taken a corrosive agent, such as lye, ammonia, or mineral acids. Bringing any of these agents back up the patient's esophagus will cause further damage. Instead, quickly neutralize their acidity with the appropriate antidote, and care for the patient according to the doctor's instructions.

Performing a gastric lavage requires this equipment: a large irrigating syringe or bulb syringe, 120 to 500 ml of tap water or normal saline solution (100 ml if your patient's a child), two basins, a suctioning machine, and the proper antidote, as ordered by the doctor. (For a list of proper antidotes to use for specific poisons, see the chart on page 120.)

Gastric intubation and lavage

Performing a gastric lavage continued

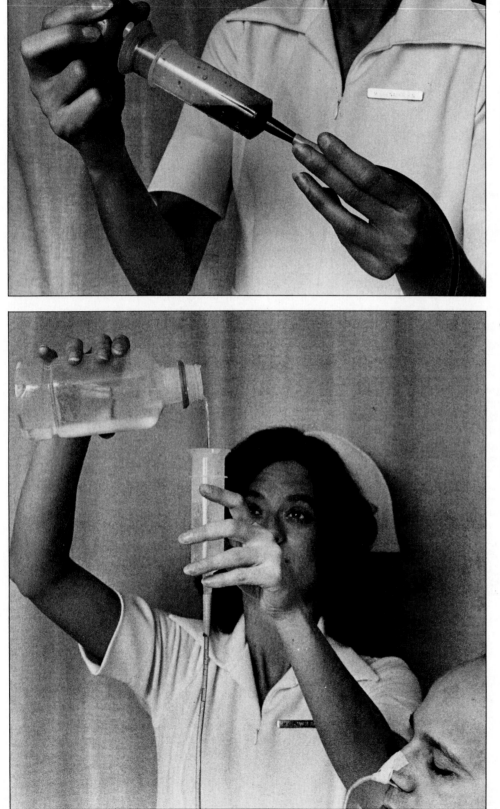

2 Place your patient in the high Fowler's position (or as ordered by the doctor) for this procedure. *Note:* A severely combative patient may try to pull out his nasogastric tube. Get orders from the doctor to restrain him.

Check for correct placement of the nasogastric tube. Then, attach the syringe to the tube, as shown here. Aspirate the patient's stomach contents, and empty it into one of the basins. Put it aside for laboratory analysis.

3 Then, remove the bulb or plunger from the syringe. Elevate the end of the tubing above your patient's head.

Slowly pour up to 500 ml water or normal saline solution into the tube. To avoid overfilling the patient's stomach, watch for signs of stomach distention or vomiting. *Important:* If your patient begins to vomit, stop instillation immediately, and turn his head to one side. Allow the nasogastric tube to drain, and then suction your patient's mouth and trachea. Make sure his airway is open.

4 Now, position the unused basin next to the patient. Remove the syringe barrel from the tube. Place the end of the tube into the basin, and let the gravitational pull siphon your patient's stomach contents. Repeat the entire procedure at least 10 times, or until the fluid withdrawn from his stomach becomes clear.

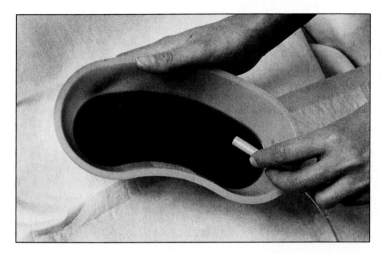

5 When you've finished the gastric lavage, the doctor will want you to do one of the following: instill proper antidote; position tube for gravitational drainage; temporarily clamp tube closed; attach tube to suctioning machine for intermittent suction; or remove tube entirely.

Important: Does your hospital's policy require that you send aspirated stomach contents to the lab for analysis? If so, pour contents into a container labeled with the patient's name, hospital identification number, time and date. Never discard stomach contents in suspected drug overdose cases before checking hospital policy.

Document everything in your nurses' notes.

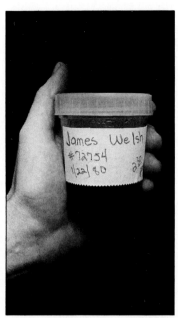

Performing an iced gastric lavage

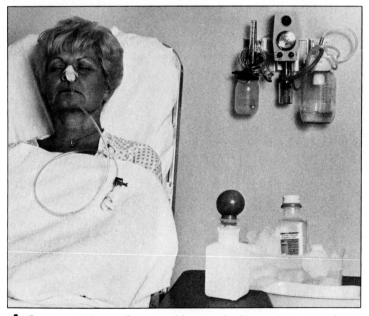

1 *On page 111 you discovered how to do the most common type of gastric lavage. But suppose the doctor wants you to perform a gastric lavage with iced saline solution. Would you know how? This kind of lavage is commonly ordered for patients with GI bleeding. To do this procedure properly, follow these instructions:*

First, gather your equipment: a 60 cc syringe, a 500 ml bottle of normal saline solution, a sterile bowl, an emesis basin, and a basin filled with ice.

Put your patient in a high Fowler's position, and check placement of her nasogastric tube, using the guidelines on page 111. Put the bottle of saline solution in the basin of ice. Cool solution to approximately 30° F. (−1.1° C.). Then, pour it into the sterile bowl.

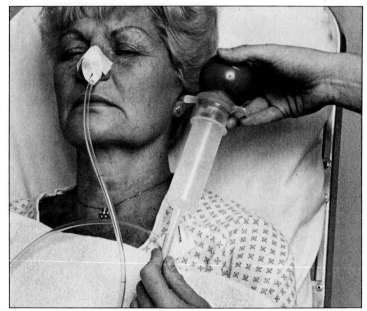

2 Fill the 60 cc syringe with the iced saline solution. Then, attach the syringe to the nasogastric tube, as shown here. Instill the saline solution into the tube. Wait for at least 1 minute. Then, withdraw the fluid back into the syringe. If resistance is met, allow the tube to drain by gravity into the emesis basin. Put the withdrawn fluid into a container. Repeat the procedure until all the withdrawn fluid is relatively clear, or as ordered. You may need *more* than 500 ml of solution. Measure the fluid in the container, and document the amount and color—as well as the entire procedure—in your nurses' notes.

Cardiovascular emergencies

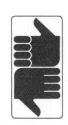

When to use rotating tourniquets

As you probably know, rotating tourniquet therapy is sometimes used to help patients who have severe lung congestion. How does it work? Special tourniquet cuffs are simultaneously applied to three of the patient's extremities. The applied pressure pools blood in those extremities, which, in turn, decreases venous blood return to the patient's heart.

• The doctor *may* order rotating tourniquets for a patient suffering from congestive heart failure or acute pulmonary edema. But first, he will have attempted (and failed) to help the patient with other methods of treatment; for example, potent diuretic therapy, digitalis therapy, or possibly a phlebotomy.

• The doctor *won't* order rotating tourniquets if the patient has any circulatory problems, is in hypovolemic shock, or has a preexisting infection or ischemia.

Applying rotating tourniquets

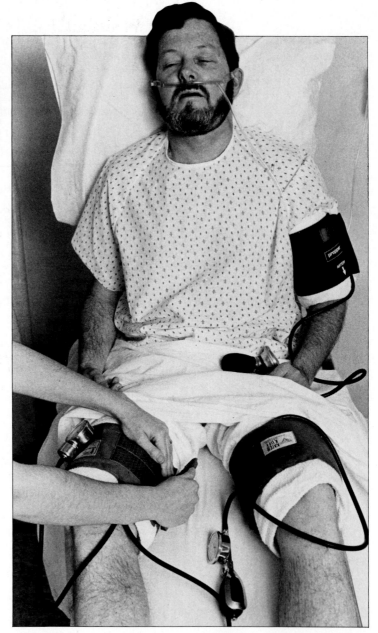

1 *Let's assume your patient has acute pulmonary edema and hasn't responded to potent diuretics. In such a case, the doctor will probably order rotating tourniquets. Use an automatic rotating tourniquet machine (Danzer apparatus) for this therapy. But if your hospital doesn't have one—or it's already in use—you may have to apply blood pressure cuffs to perform this procedure. Here's how:*

First, gather your equipment. The nurse shown here has decided to use three cuffs. Some nurses use four, leaving one cuff uninflated at all times. Explain the procedure and its purpose to your patient. Prepare him for the possibility that the cuff pressure may temporarily make his arms and legs appear cyanotic.

Then, record his blood pressure, apical heart rate, radial and pedal pulses, and respiration rate for baseline data reference.

2 Now you're ready to apply the cuffs. Wrap a small towel or washcloth as high as possible around each arm and leg. Then, apply the cuffs directly over this padding, as the nurse is doing here. However, don't inflate the cuffs yet.

Save $2.00 off each NURSING PHOTOBOOK

Choose your first book. Examine it for 10 days FREE!

Subscribe to the NURSING PHOTOBOOK series and save $2.00 on every volume. That's a significant savings on the entire series. And now you can select your own introductory volume from the books shown or listed.

The NURSING PHOTOBOOK series

Aiding Ambulatory Patients • Assessing Your Patients • Attending Ob/Gyn Patients • Caring for Surgical Patients • Carrying Out Special Procedures • Controlling Infection • Coping with Neurologic Disorders • Dealing with Emergencies • Ensuring Intensive Care • Giving Cardiac Care • Giving Medications • Helping Geriatric Patients • Implementing Urologic Procedures • Managing I.V. Therapy • Nursing Pediatric Patients • Performing GI Procedures • Providing Early Mobility • Providing Respiratory Care • Using Monitors • Working with Orthopedic Patients

This is your order card. Send no money.

Please send me _____
for a 10-day, free examination. If I decide to keep this introductory volume, I agree to pay $14.95, plus shipping and handling. I understand that I will receive another PHOTOBOOK approximately every other month, each on the same 10-day, free-examination basis. There is no minimum number of books I must buy, and I may cancel my subscription at any time simply by notifying you.

G5-PB

I don't want the series. Just send me _____.
I will pay $16.95 for each copy, plus shipping and handling. Please send me _____ copies and bill me.

G5-SP

Name _____

Address _____

City _____ State _____ Zip _____

Price subject to change. Offer valid in U.S. only.

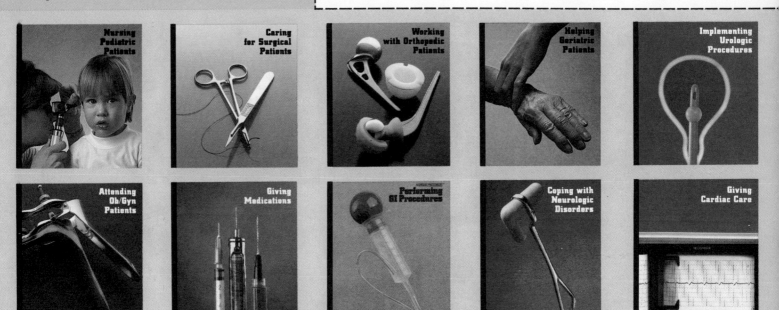

© 1983 Intermed Communications, Inc.

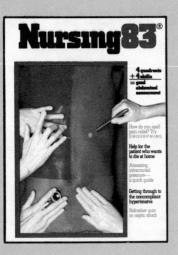

GET ACQUAINTED WITH THE WORLD'S LARGEST NURSING JOURNAL TODAY!

Mail the postage-paid card at right. ▶

Keep your nursing skills growing... with *Nursing83.*

Keep up to date on the latest breakthroughs in nursing care every month in **Nursing83.** With **Nursing83,** you'll be the first to learn about the new techniques and procedures that will mean more skills and knowledge for you... better care for your patients. All in a magazine that's easy to read, easy to understand, and colorfully illustrated to show *you* how to improve your nursing care.

☐ Send me 1 year (12 issues) of **Nursing83.** My check for $16 is enclosed, saving me $4 off the regular $20 price.

☐ Please bill me later for $16.

Name _____

Address _____

City _____ State _____ Zip _____

I am an: ☐ RN ☐ LPN ☐ Other   Do you work in a hospital? ☐ Yes ☐ No

7P83

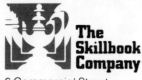
Introduce yourself to the brand-new NURSING PHOTOBOOK™ series

…the remarkable breakthrough in nursing education that can change your career. Each book in this unique series contains detailed *Photostories*… and tables, charts, and graphs to help you learn important new procedures. And each handsome PHOTOBOOK offers you ● 160 illustrated, fact-filled pages ● brilliant, high-contrast photographs ● convenient 9"x10½" size ● durable, hardcover binding ● carefully chosen bibliography ● complete index. Watch the experts at work showing you how to… administer drugs… teach your patient about his illness and its treatment… minimize trauma… understand doctors' diagnoses… increase patient comfort… and much more. Discover how you can become a better nurse by joining this exciting new series. You can examine each PHOTOBOOK at your leisure… for 10 days *absolutely free!*

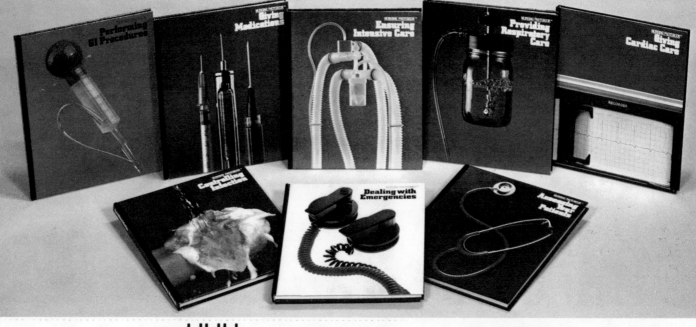

Be sure to mail the postage-paid card at left to reserve *your* first copy of *Nursing83*.

Nursing83 gives you clear, concise instruction in "hands-on" nursing. Every issue brings you in-depth clinical articles about the newest developments in nursing care—what's being discovered, researched, treated, cured. You'll learn about the new procedures, new techniques, new medications, and new equipment that will mean more skills and knowledge for you…better care for your patients!

Order your subscription today!

3 Instead, make sure you haven't applied them too tightly. To check, try to slip two fingers between the cuff and the padding. If your fingers don't slide in easily, the cuff's probably too tight. Loosen it.

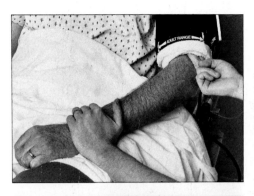

4 Inflate all the cuffs to a pressure that's less than the patient's systolic blood pressure (use your baseline data). Take care not to inflate the cuffs so tightly that you cut off arterial circulation. To check, feel for an arterial pulse in each arm and leg (distal to the cuff).

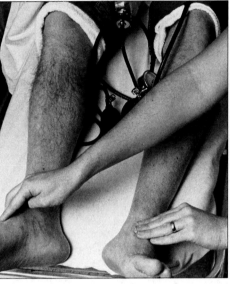

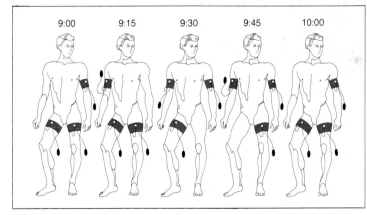

5 Rotate the cuffs every 15 minutes, using a predetermined plan such as the one illustrated here. Post the plan at your patient's bedside, and make sure it's followed. But before you proceed, be familiar with your hospital's policy regarding rotating tourniquet cuffs. Some hospitals require that all cuffs be completely removed, then reapplied, with each rotation.

After rotation, inflate the cuffs according to the guidelines already described.

If your patient's elderly or has poor peripheral circulation, rotate the cuffs every 5 minutes.

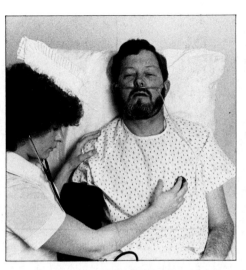

6 After each rotation, check your patient's blood pressure, as well as his heart and lung sounds. If you find any new irregularities, call the doctor at once.

In between rotations, check for adequate pulses in your patient's arms and legs. This will give you continuing assurance that the cuffs aren't inflated too tightly.

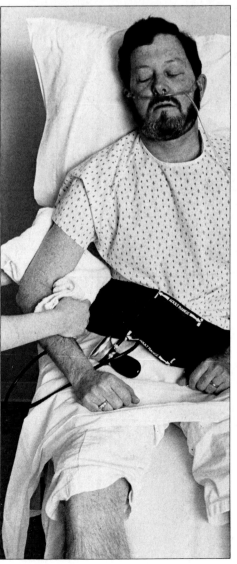

7 To discontinue the therapy, release and remove one cuff at a time (in a clockwise motion) at 15-minute intervals. Removing the cuffs in this manner prevents a sudden increase in the patient's venous blood volume, which could cause a circulatory overload.

Check your patient's blood pressure and respiration rate after each cuff is removed. If he develops respiratory distress or has a significant change in blood pressure, notify the doctor immediately. Let him tell you whether or not to remove any of the remaining cuffs.

Cardiovascular emergencies

Applying antiembolism stockings

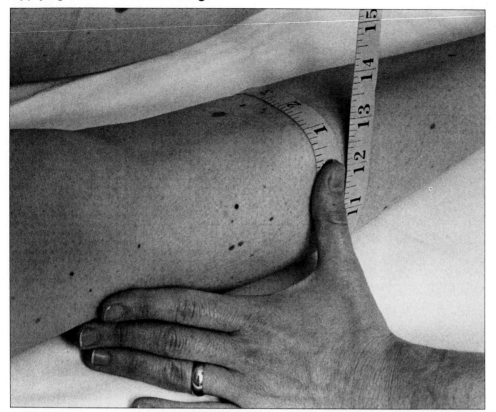

1 *Anytime a patient with a history of cardiac or venous system disorders arrives in the ED, the doctor may want you to fit her with antiembolism (elastic) stockings. Why? Because antiembolism stockings compress superficial veins and force blood into the deep veins, minimizing the risk of thrombus formation. When these stockings are fitted correctly, they also keep blood from pooling in the patient's legs, thereby increasing the venous blood return to her heart.*

Here's how to apply them: Begin by determining the proper size stocking for your patient. First, measure the largest part of her calf, as she lies flat on her back.

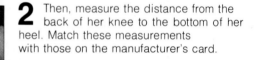

2 Then, measure the distance from the back of her knee to the bottom of her heel. Match these measurements with those on the manufacturer's card.

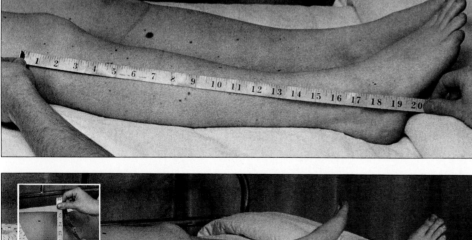

3 Did the doctor order thigh- or waist-length stockings? Instead of measuring from the patient's knee to her heel, measure all the way from her gluteal furrow, as shown here. [Inset] Also measure the largest part of her thigh.

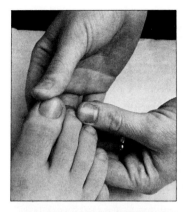

4 Before applying the stocking, check the color, sensation, and motor function in each of your patient's legs. If her legs appear cool or cyanotic, notify the doctor before proceeding.

Make sure your patient's legs are clean and dry. If you must cleanse the patient's legs, don't rub her calves. Doing so could dislodge an embolus.

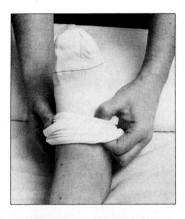

5 To apply the stockings, roll down the stocking top to the heel. Then, pull the stocking over your patient's foot, as shown here.

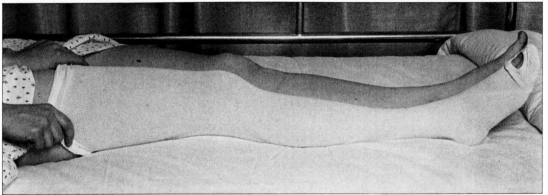

6 Once the heel is in place, unroll the rest of the stocking over the patient's leg, as the nurse is doing here. If you're applying waist-length stockings, make sure you also fit your patient with an adjustable waist belt. Attach the stockings to the belt, but take care that the side panels and waistband aren't pressing against a catheter, a drainage tube, or an incision.

7 Never apply stockings that seem too tight. Doing so could constrict the patient's circulation. As a safeguard, pull on the toes of the stockings to make sure they're not exerting excessive pressure. Remove the stockings at least once each shift, and check skin color, sensation, circulation, and movement in the patient's legs. Notify the doctor if your patient complains of leg pain, has dusky-colored toenail beds, decreased or absent pedal pulses, or reddened areas. Document your findings on her chart.

Cardiovascular emergencies

How to apply warm, moist compresses

1 *If your patient develops phlebitis in her leg from prolonged bedrest or I.V. therapy, she runs the risk of the embolus migrating to a coronary artery. To minimize this risk, the doctor may want you to apply warm, moist compresses. Here's how:*

First, place a plastic square or bedsaver pad under your patient's affected leg. Then, place a bath blanket directly on top of the plastic.

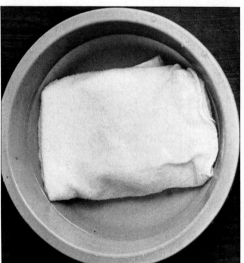

2 Depending on your patient's leg size, obtain a clean towel, washcloth, or large piece of gauze. At her bedside, soak the cloth in water that's been warmed to about 105° F. (40.6° C.), never hotter. Wring out the excess moisture.

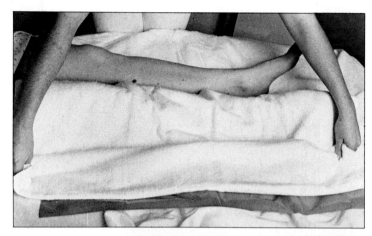

3 Ask the patient to raise her leg. Then, place the moist compress on the affected area, along the vein's pathway. When you do, take care not to rub the area or you could dislodge the embolus.

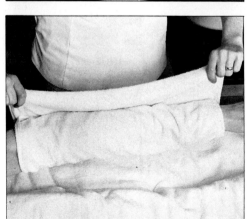

4 Gently but quickly, position the leg flat against the bath blanket. Cover the leg immediately by drawing up the edges of the plastic square, as shown here.

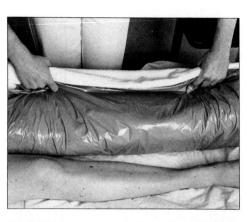

5 Next, tape the plastic to hold it in place.
☛ *Nursing tip:* If your patient's a child, you may want to further secure the plastic by covering it with a stockinette or a large cotton sock.

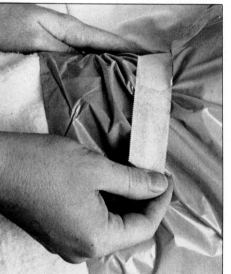

6 At least once every 15 to 20 minutes, remove the tape and plastic covering, and check the compress' temperature. Also, check the patient's skin for possible irritation. When the compress begins to cool, replace it immediately with a new one, using the procedure outlined above.

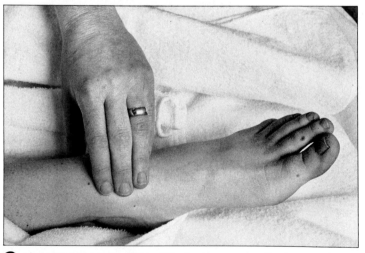

Using a disposable electric K-pad

1 *To provide continuous warmth without having to replace moist compresses, use a disposable electric K-pad, such as the one shown here.* The K-pad, which is placed *over* the taped plastic covering, works similarly to an electric heating pad, except it has hot water circulating through its internal coils.

If you decide to use a K-pad, make sure you also obtain the water reservoir that accompanies it.

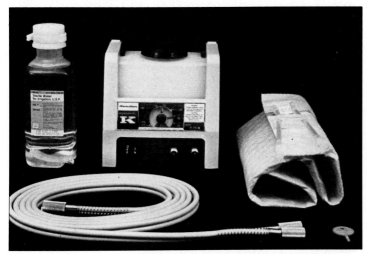

2 Follow these instructions for applying the K-pad: First, use distilled water to fill the reservoir to the proper level.

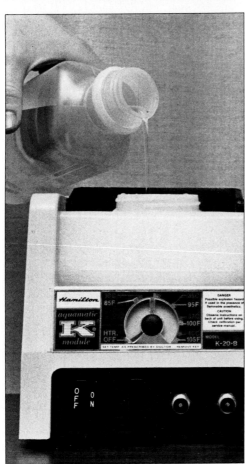

3 Attach the water reservoir tubing to the disposable K-pad, as shown here. [Inset] Make sure the connection is secure.

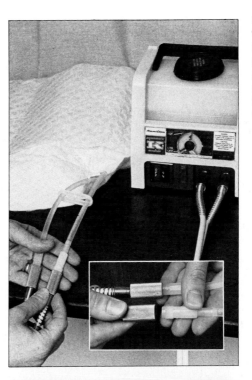

4 Then, plug the unit into an electrical outlet. Use the key provided with the unit to set the correct temperature, as ordered by the doctor. Allow at least 1½ minutes for it to heat.

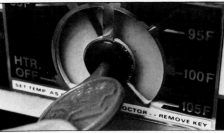

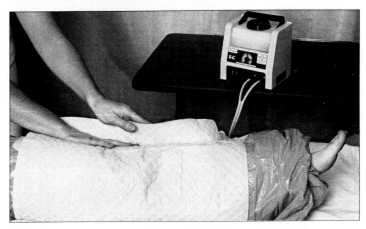

5 Place the K-pad *over* the taped plastic covering on the patient's affected leg. Never place it directly over the compress. Keep the water reservoir at the same level as the pad or above it. Refill the reservoir, if needed.

Remember, when your patient no longer needs moist compresses, you can discard the disposable K-pad. However, save the water reservoir for use with another pad.

Systemic emergencies

National Poison Center Network ® Poison Treatment Chart

How to use this chart
Locate the substance that has poisoned your patient in the columns below. The number listed after the poison corresponds with the appropriate treatment in the management columns listed to the right.

Suggested general treatment for poisoning management

1
There should be no problem in small amounts.
No treatment necessary.
Fluids may be given.

2
Induce vomiting. Give syrup of ipecac in the following dosages:
Under 1 year of age:
Two teaspoons followed by at least 2 to 3 glasses of liquid.
One year and over:
Give 1 tablespoon followed by at least 2 to 3 glasses of liquid.
Do not induce vomiting if the patient is semicomatose, comatose, or convulsing.
Call Poison Center for additional information.

3
Dilute or neutralize with water or milk. **Do not induce vomiting.** Gastric lavage is indicated. Call Poison Center for specific instructions.

4
Treat symptomatically unless botulism is suspected. Call Poison Center for specific information regarding botulism.

A
Acetone 2
Acids
  Ingestion 5
  Eye contamination 7
  Topical 6
  Inhalation if mixed with
  bleach 9
Aerosols
  Eye contamination 7
  Inhalation 9
After-shave lotions (see Cologne)
Airplane glue 10
Alcohol
  Ingestion 2
  Eye contamination 7
Ammonia
  Ingestion 5
  Eye contamination 7
  Inhalation 9
Amphetamine 2, 8
Analgesics 10
Aniline dyes
  Ingestion 2, 8
  Inhalation 8, 9
  Topical 6, 8
Antacids 1
Antibiotics
  Less than 2 to 3 times total
  daily dose 1
  More than 3 times total daily
  dose 2
Antidepressants
  Tricyclic 2, 8
  Others 2
Antifreeze (ethylene glycol)
  Ingestion 2
  Eye contamination 7
Antihistamines 2, 8
Antiseptics 2
Ant trap
  Kepone type 1

Others 2
Aquarium products 1
Arsenic 2, 8
Aspirin 2

B
Baby oil 1
Ball-point ink 1
Barbiturates
  Short-acting 10
  Long-acting 2
Bathroom bowl cleaner
  Ingestion 5
  Eye contamination 7
  Inhalation if mixed with
  bleach 9
  Topical 6
Batteries
  Dry cell (flashlight) 1
  Mercury (hearing aid) 2
  Wet cell (automobile) 5
Benzene
  Ingestion 10
  Inhalation 9
  Topical 6
Birth control pills 1
Bleaches
  Liquid ingestion 1
  Solid ingestion 5
  Eye contamination 7
  Inhalation when mixed with
  acids or alkalies 9
Boric acid 2
Bromides 2
Bubble bath 1

C
Camphor 2
Candles 1

Caps
  Less than one roll 1
  More than one roll 2
Carbon monoxide 9
Carbon tetrachloride
  Ingestion 2
  Inhalation 9
  Topical 6
Chalk 1
Chlorine bleach (see Bleaches)
Cigarettes
  Less than one 1
  One or more 2
Clay 1
Cleaning fluids 10
Cleanser (household) 1
Clinitest tablets 5
Cold remedies 10
Cologne
  Less than 15 ml 1
  More than 15 ml 2
Contraceptive pills 1
Corn/wart removers 5
Cosmetics (see specific type)
Cough medicines 10
Crayons
  Children's 1
  Others 2
Cyanide 8

D
Dandruff shampoo 2
Dehumidifying packets 1
Denture adhesives 1
Denture cleansers 5
Deodorants
  All types 1
Deodorizer cakes 2
Deodorizers, room 10
Desiccants 1
Detergents
  Liquid/powder (general) ... 1

Electric dishwasher and phosphate-free 5
Diaper rash ointment 1
Dishwasher detergents (see Detergents)
Disinfectants 3
Drain cleaners (see Lye)
Dyes
  Aniline (see Aniline dyes)
  Others 2

E
Electric dishwasher detergent (see Detergents)
Epoxy glue
  Catalyst 5
  Resin or when mixed 10
Epsom salts 2
Ethyl alcohol (see Alcohol)
Ethylene glycol (see Antifreeze)
Eye makeup 1

F
Fabric softeners 2
Fertilizers 10
Fishbowl additives 1
Food poisoning 4
Furniture polish 10

G
Gas (natural) 9
Gasoline 10
Glue 10
Gun products 10

H
Hair dyes
  Ingestion 3
  Eye contamination 7
  Topical 6

Courtesy Richard W. Moriarty, MD, Director, National Poison Center Network, Children's Hospital of Pittsburgh

5

Dilute or neutralize with water or milk. **Do not induce vomiting.** Gastric lavage should be avoided. This substance may cause burns of the mucous membranes. Consult ENT specialist following emergency treatment. Call Poison Center for specific information.

6

Immediately wash skin thoroughly with running water. Call Poison Center for further treatment.

7

Immediately wash eyes with a gentle stream of running water. Continue for 15 minutes. Call Poison Center for further treatment.

8

Specific antagonist may be indicated. Call Poison Center.

9

Remove patient to fresh air. Support respirations. Call Poison Center for further treatment.

10

Call Poison Center for specific instructions.

11

Symptomatic and supportive treatment. **Do not induce vomiting for ingestion.** Give naloxone hydrochloride (Narcan*) I.V. as indicated for respiratory depression.
Dosage:
Adult—0.4 mg I.V.
  May be repeated at 2- to 3- minute intervals.
Child—0.01 mg/kg I.V.
  May be repeated at 5- to 10-minute intervals.

*Available in the United States and in Canada.

Systemic emergencies

Coping with anaphylactic shock

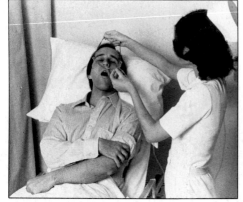

1 *Grady Morrison, a 20-year-old house painter, is rushed to the ED with a wasp sting on his forearm. You see at once that he's having trouble breathing, his eyes are puffy, and his arm is swollen. Experience tells you that Grady has gone into anaphylactic shock. Do you know what to do?*

First, check for an open airway. If your patient develops a sudden airway obstruction from laryngeal edema, be ready to assist the doctor with an endotracheal intubation. Or, have an emergency trach tray handy in case the doctor has to perform a tracheotomy (see page 26). If the doctor isn't immediately available, be prepared to do an emergency cricothyreotomy (see page 25).

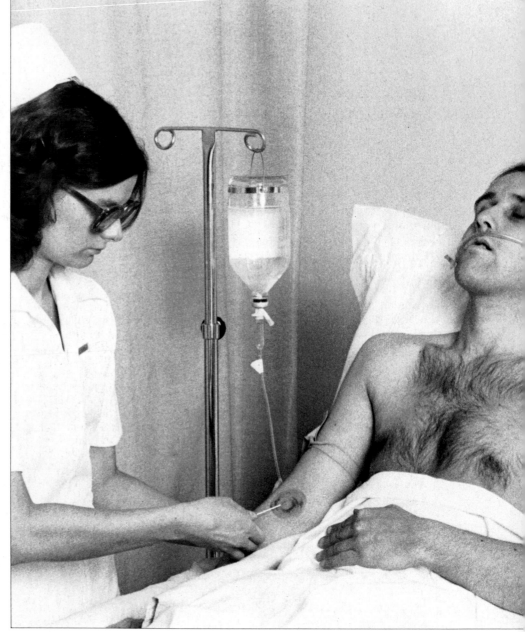

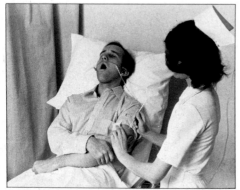

2 Next, administer epinephrine hydrochloride (Adrenalin*) 0.3 to 0.5 ml I.M. or subcutaneously, as ordered by the doctor. Then, vigorously massage the injection site to increase absorption. Repeat the dose every 3 to 5 minutes, administering four to five doses.

Now, give an antihistamine, such as diphenhydramine hydrochloride (Benadryl*), 50 to 100 mg orally, I.M., or I.V. (depending on the patient's condition, size, and age). This drug, given in combination with epinephrine, may be all the treatment Grady will need.

3 But, if his shock signs and symptoms continue, start an I.V. with lactated Ringer's solution, using a large-bore catheter. Check Grady's blood pressure at regular intervals. If you notice a sudden drop in his blood pressure, administer a vasopressor, like levarterenol (Levophed*) or dopamine (Intropin*), by I.V. infusion to constrict the vessels, as ordered by the doctor. Remember to watch the injection site for signs of drug infiltration; for example, redness and swelling. If you see any of these signs, stop the I.V. immediately. Notify the doctor.

Fortunately, you can almost always reverse anaphylactic shock with prompt, effective action. But your responsibility doesn't end there. Warn Grady to take precautions not to get stung again. But, remind him that if he does, he can administer the anaphylactic drug himself with the kit shown on the opposite page. Show him how to use it.

Encourage Grady to carry identification that will advise others of his potential for severe allergic reactions; for example, Medic Alert jewelry, as shown on page 15.

*Available in the United States and in Canada.

Patient teaching

How to use an anaphylaxis kit

1 Dear Patient:
Because you risk having a severe reaction from an insect sting or other antigen, the doctor has given you this emergency anaphylaxis kit. Everything you need to combat the allergic reaction is inside: a prefilled syringe containing two doses of epinephrine, alcohol swabs, a tourniquet, and Chlo-Amine (antihistamine) tablets.

If you're stung by an insect—despite precautions—use the kit as follows. Also, notify the doctor immediately, or ask someone else to call him.

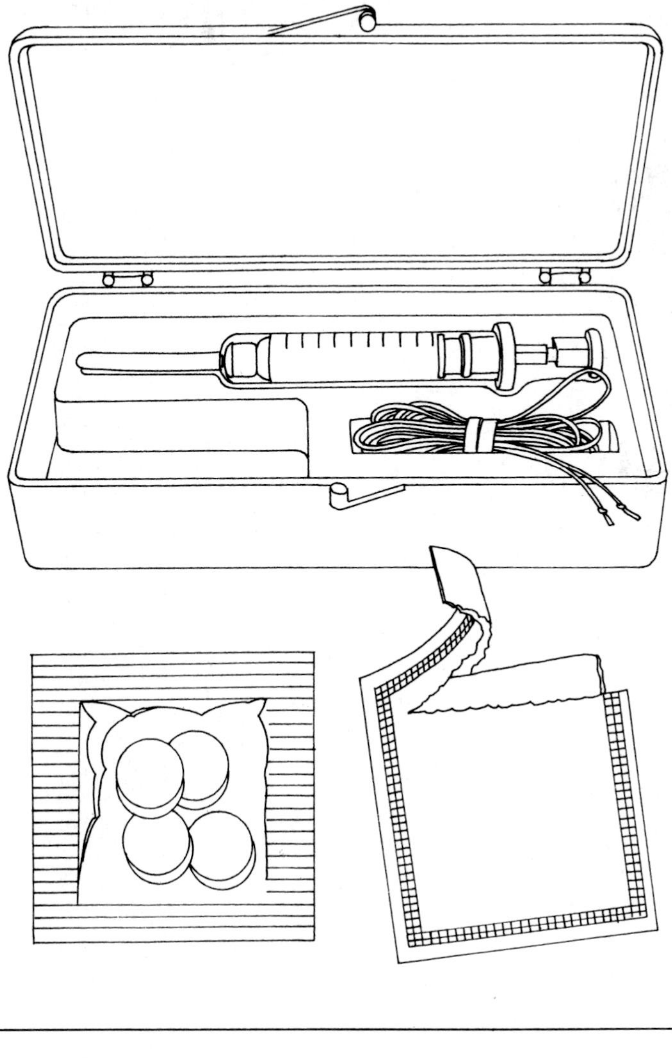

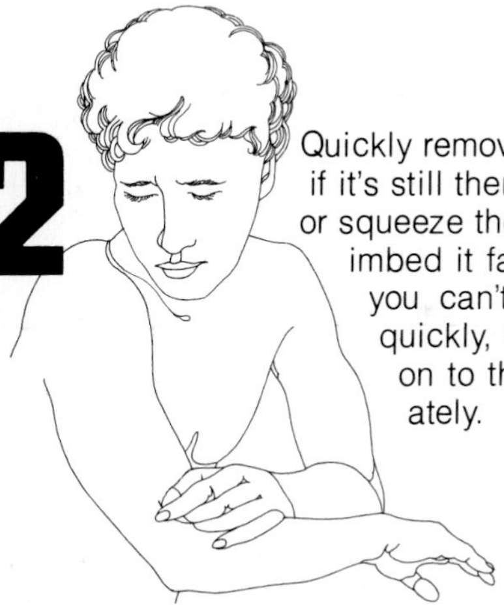

2 Quickly remove the insect's stinger if it's still there. Don't pinch, push, or squeeze the stinger, as you may imbed it farther into the skin. If you can't remove the stinger quickly, don't keep trying. Go on to the next step immediately.

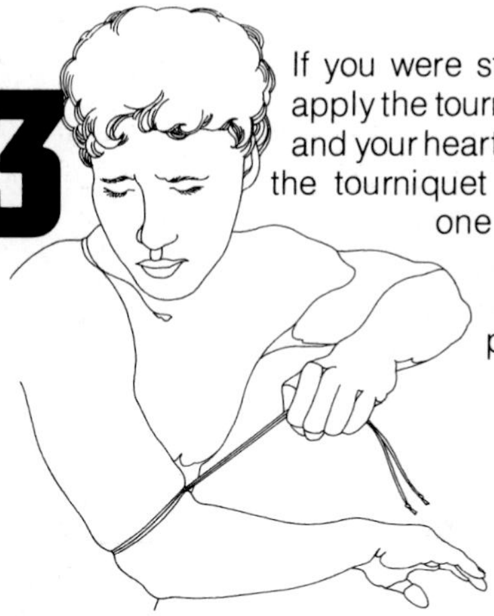

3 If you were stung on an arm or leg, apply the tourniquet between the sting and your heart, as shown here. Tighten the tourniquet by pulling the end of one string. Remember to release the tourniquet after 10 minutes by pulling on the metal ring.

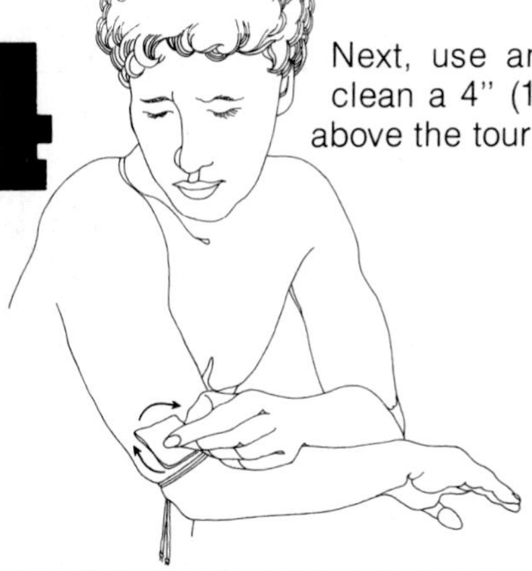

4 Next, use an alcohol swab to clean a 4" (10 cm) area of skin above the tourniquet.

Patient teaching

How to use an anaphylaxis kit continued

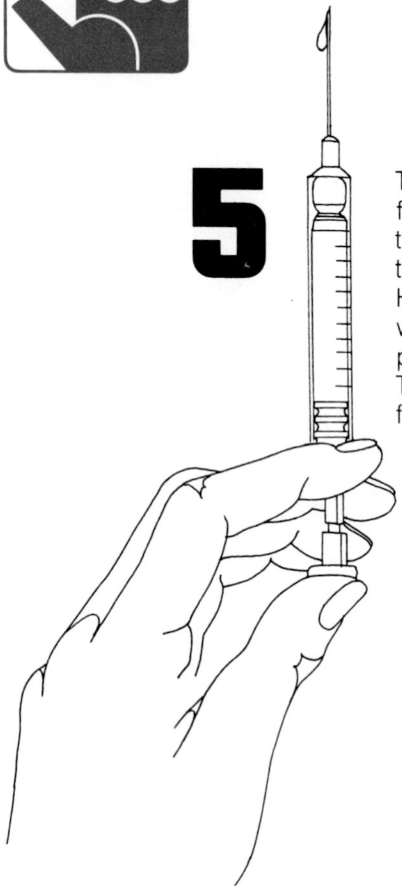

5 Then, lift the pre-filled syringe from the kit, and remove the needle cover. Hold the syringe with the needle pointing upward. Then, expel any air from it by carefully pushing on the plunger, as shown here.

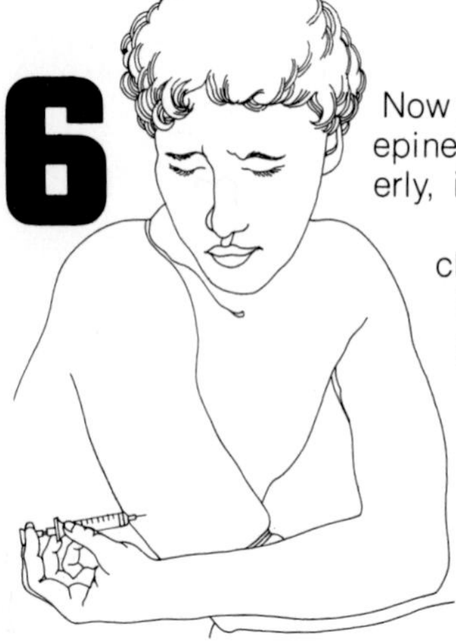

6 Now you're ready to inject the epinephrine. To do this properly, insert the entire needle straight down into the cleansed skin. Then, pull back slightly on the plunger. If you see blood in the syringe, the needle's inside a blood vessel. Withdraw the needle, and reinsert it in another site.

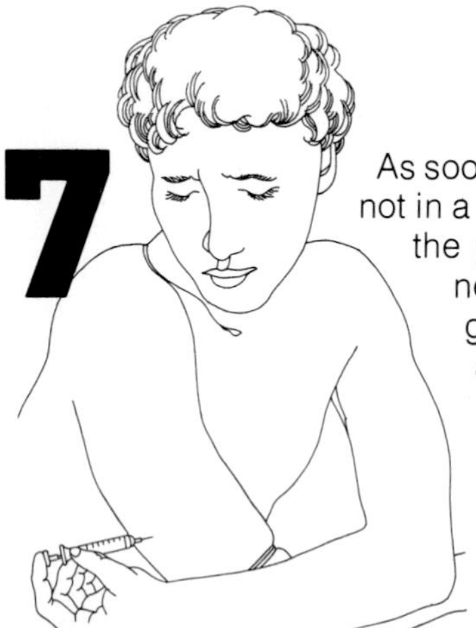

7 As soon as you're sure the needle's not in a blood vessel, push down on the plunger, and inject the epinephrine. Use the following guidelines for proper dosage: *adults, and children (over age 12):* 0.01 to 0.5 ml; *children (between ages 7 and 12):* 0.2 ml; *children (between ages 2 and 6):* 0.15 ml.

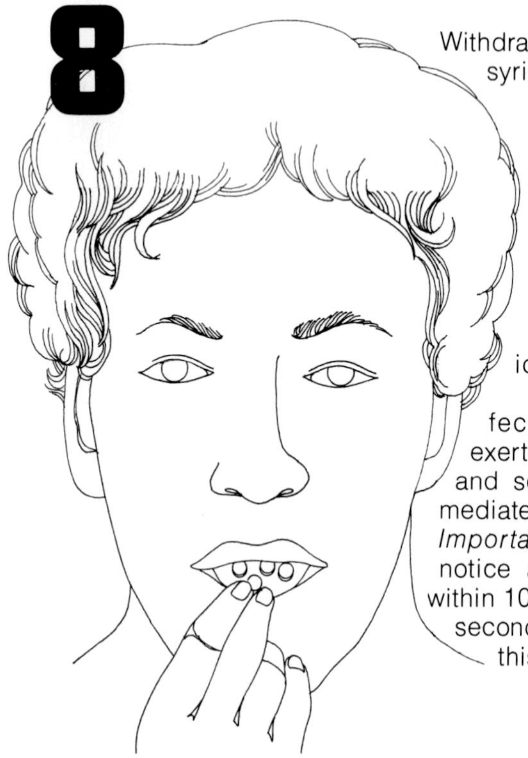

8 Withdraw the needle and syringe. Then, chew and swallow the Chlo-Amine tablets. If you're over age 12, take four tablets; if you're under age 12, take two tablets.

Next, apply ice packs, if available, to the affected area. Avoid exertion, keep warm, and see a doctor immediately.

Important: If you don't notice an improvement within 10 minutes, give a second injection. To do this, rotate the rectangular plunger a quarter turn to the right, and line it up with the rectangular slot in the syringe. Don't depress the plunger until you're ready to administer the second injection. Then follow the same injection procedure as before.

Some special guidelines

Nurses' guide to common nontraumatic emergencies

When you're faced with a nontraumatic emergency, how can you identify what's wrong? And how should you deal with the problem? For any nontraumatic emergency, begin by making your patient as comfortable as possible. Reassure him. Then, start an I.V. with the appropriate solution. At the same time, draw blood for lab studies. Closely monitor all vital signs. These steps will ensure that you're prepared if your patient goes into shock.

But what do you do in addition to the above? That depends on the specific emergency. The chart below will tell you what you need to know about 15 common nontraumatic emergencies. Study it.

Problem	Possible causes	Signs and symptoms	Nursing considerations
Appendicitis	• Infection of the appendix • Pinworms	• Pain in right lower abdominal quadrant, with local tenderness (McBurney's point); or periumbilical colicky pain • Muscle spasms in right and left lower abdominal quadrants • Low-grade fever: 100° to 101° F. (37.8° to 38.3° C.) • Elevated white blood cell count (WBC) • Positive psoas sign	• Follow general guidelines listed earlier. • Notify doctor. He'll perform a rectal examination, as well as a pelvic examination in females, to rule out pelvic inflammatory disease (PID). • Reassure the patient as much as possible, and explain what to expect. • Prepare the patient for surgery, as ordered by the doctor.
Bleeding esophageal varisces	• Portal hypertension from cirrhosis of the liver, or portal vein obstruction • Duodenal ulcer • Severe gastritis • Circulation abnormalities in splenic vein or superior vena cava	• History of alcoholism or portal hypertension • Severe bleeding through mouth and nose • Restlessness, agitation, apprehension • Respiratory distress from aspiration of blood • Jaundice	• Follow general guidelines listed earlier. • Assist doctor with insertion of Sengstaken-Blakemore tube, if needed. • Prepare patient for endoscopy. • Administer vitamin K intramuscularly, if the doctor orders. • Never sedate such a patient because it could cause him to lapse into a coma.
Bowel obstruction (mechanical)	• Adhesions from surgery • Hernia • Volvulus • Malignant neoplasm • Hematoma • Intussusception	• Wavelike pain or cramps in abdomen • Abdominal distention (in upper abdomen if obstruction is high in small bowel; in midabdomen if obstruction is low in small bowel; in mid- to lower abdomen if obstruction is in large intestine) • Electrolyte imbalance: metabolic alkalosis, which, if left untreated, may lead to profound dehydration and metabolic acidosis • Hyperactive bowel sounds, with possible bilious vomitus	• Follow general guidelines listed earlier. • Notify doctor. • Prepare patient for flat plate X-ray to confirm diagnosis. • Assist doctor in insertion of nasogastric tube, to relieve gastric and small bowel distention and to drain bile. • If obstruction is partly in the small bowel and partly in the large intestine, assist doctor with insertion of Miller-Abbott tube. • If obstruction is in large bowel, prepare patient for sigmoidoscopy and emergency barium enema. • Don't give patient food or liquids. • Prepare patient for surgery.
Bowel obstruction (non-mechanical: paralytic ileus)	• Back injuries • Fractures • Complication of surgery	• Nausea, vomiting • Gaseous distention • Dull or diffused pain in abdominal area • Absent bowel sounds • Dehydration	• Follow general guidelines listed earlier. • Insert Foley catheter to monitor urinary output. • Insert nasogastric tube for decompression and control of vomiting. • Start an I.V. to administer normal saline solution with KCl added. • Prepare the patient for surgery, if necessary.
Congestive heart failure	• Pulmonary embolism • Heart disease, myocarditis, MI • Anesthesia • Thyrotoxicosis • Hypertension • Stress • Pregnancy	• Fatigue • Weight gain • Tachycardia • Skin temperature, cool; skin color, dusky • Dyspnea, orthopnea, rales, cough • Neck vein distention • Liver distention • Pitting peripheral edema in the ankle and pretibial area	• Follow general guidelines listed earlier. • Place patient in a high Fowler's position. • Administer digitalis and diuretics, as ordered. • Administer oxygen. • Periodically draw arterial blood for blood gas measurements. • Apply rotating tourniquets, per doctor's orders. See page 114 for guidelines.

Some special guidelines

Nurses' guide to common nontraumatic emergencies continued

Problem	Possible causes	Signs and symptoms	Nursing considerations
Delirium tremens	• Alcohol withdrawal	• Severe psychomotor agitation, confusion, disorientation • Visual and auditory hallucinations • Dilated pupils, fever, tachycardia, profuse sweating • Elevated vital signs • Generalized seizures, usually grand mal • Combativeness • History of alcohol abuse	• Follow general guidelines listed earlier. • Administer adequate sedation, as ordered, to relieve CNS irritability. For example, the doctor may order chlordiazepoxide (Librium*), 50 to 100 mg I.M.; chlorpromazine hydrochloride (Thorazine), 100 mg I.M.; or paraldehyde, 5 ml I.M. or 4 to 10 ml orally. To improve taste of medication, mix it with juice. ▱ *Nursing tip:* Paraldehyde reacts with some plastics, so administer it in a glass syringe. • Put patient in private room, if possible, and keep it well lighted to reduce visual hallucinations. • Maintain patient's fluid and electrolyte balance. Make sure I.V. solutions contain vitamin supplement. Or give vitamins orally. • Control nausea and vomiting to prevent massive GI bleeding or esophageal rupture. • Apply protective restraints, if ordered by doctor. • Reassure patient that his hallucinations will stop when he's completed withdrawal. • Tape a padded tongue depressor to the patient's bed in case of seizure. • Refer patient and family to social service.
Diabetic ketoacidosis (hyperglycemia)	• Acute insulin deficiency	• Early symptoms include thirst; vomiting; abdominal pain; visual disturbances; dizziness; weakness; headache; restlessness; dry, hot, flushed skin. • Later symptoms include lethargy, possible coma, Kussmaul's respiration, fruity breath, hypotension. • Blood test shows elevated glucose level and plasma ketones • ABG's show decreased CO_2 • Glycosuria, with possible ketones	• Follow general guidelines listed earlier. • Test urine for presence of ketones and glucose level. • Administer a regular insulin, either subcutaneously or intravenously, as ordered by doctor. • Give half- or full-strength normal saline solution or lactated Ringer's solution, following doctor's orders, to correct electrolyte imbalance. • Maintain an accurate intake and output record. • Insert Foley catheter, if ordered.
Drug overdose	• Excessive drug ingestion	• History of drug abuse • Depending on drug, patient may have respiratory depression; cold and clammy skin; lethargy; dilated or constricted pupils; weak, rapid pulse; decreased or increased tendon reflexes; coma; agitation; arrhythmias; hallucinations.	• Follow general guidelines listed earlier. • Insert Foley catheter, if ordered. • Insert NG tube to remove stomach contents (if drug was ingested). Save contents for lab analysis. Prepare for gastric lavage, if ordered. • Administer narcotic antagonist naloxone hydrochloride (Narcan*), as ordered. • Draw arterial blood sample to obtain ABGs.
Evisceration	• Improper healing of incision, possibly from circulatory or pulmonary difficulties • Penetrating trauma	• Visible separation of incision (or wound) edges (dehiscence), permitting viscera to protrude • Local pain • Possible bleeding at site • History of recent abdominal surgery or penetrating trauma	• Follow general guidelines listed earlier. • Instruct patient to remain in bed. • Have someone notify the doctor at once. • Immediately apply sterile dressings soaked in normal saline solution directly over the evisceration. *Caution:* Never probe or attempt to force protruding viscera back into the abdominal cavity. • Prepare the patient for surgery.
Gastrointestinal bleeding	• Peptic ulcer • Gastritis • Malignant neoplasm • Diverticulitis • Ulcerative colitis • Hemorrhoids	• Blood pressure decreasing, pulse rate increasing • Hematemesis and/or melena • Vomitus looks like coffee grounds • Abdominal tenderness and distension • Pale skin color • Fatigue • Hyperperistalsis • Blood test shows decreased hemoglobin and hematocrit.	• Follow general guidelines listed earlier. • Insert nasogastric tube, and perform iced gastric lavage, if ordered (see pages 106 and 113). • Administer oxygen. • Prepare patient for gastroscopy. • Draw blood for type and crossmatch. • Check patient's stool and vomitus for occult blood.

Problem	Possible causes	Signs and symptoms	Nursing considerations
Hypertensive crisis	• Renal disease (acute or chronic), chronic pyelone-phritis, or renal vascular disease • Pheochromocytoma • MAO inhibitor drug therapy • Acute cardiac insuffi-ciency • Intracranial hemor-rhage • Acute dissecting aneu-rysm	• High blood pressure (diastolic between 130 and 140) • Blurred vision • Severe headache • Bleeding from nose • Numbness in fingers and toes • Lethargy or semicomatose • History of hypertension	• Follow general guidelines listed earlier. • Be ready to assist doctor with insertion of arterial line for continuous blood pressure monitoring. • Be ready to administer prescribed medications; for example, furosemide (Lasix*), methyldopa (Aldomet*), or nitroprusside sodium (Nipride*). *Important:* These drugs must be administered intra-venously. • Insert a Foley catheter, if ordered.
Insulin shock (hypoglycemia)	• Glucose deprivation	• If patient's blood sugar level's between 50 and 70 mg per 100 ml of blood, he may have diaphoresis, confusion, headache, and dizziness. • If it's between 40 and 50 mg per 100 ml of blood, he may have disori-entation, tachycardia, convulsions, or coma.	• Follow general guidelines listed earlier. • Get glucose level, if possible. • Give appropriate I.V. fluid, as ordered. • To help a conscious patient, give some form of sugar orally, or glucagon (1 mg for adult) either I.M. or subcutaneously, as ordered. *Important:* Never give oral medications, food, or liquid to an uncon-scious patient.
Pulmonary edema	• Cardiac disease, in-cluding left ventricular heart failure, chronic heart failure, and mitral valve disease • Circulatory overload • Injury to central ner-vous system • Infection, fever	• Severe dyspnea, orthopnea, coughing • Pallor, diaphoresis, tachycardia • Frothy sputum (white or pink) • Widely dispersed rales • S_3 or S_4 heart sounds • Restless sleep	• Follow general guidelines listed earlier. • Place patient in high Fowler's position. • Attach patient to cardiac monitor. • Insert Foley catheter; record output ½ hourly. • Give high-flow oxygen by facemask or nasal cannula, depending on ABG measurements. • As ordered, give a potent diuretic I.V. • As ordered, give morphine to relieve agitation. • In severe cases, if ordered, apply rotating tourni-quets, following the procedure on page 114. • Perform phlebotomy, as ordered, to decrease circulating blood volume. • Per orders, give a fast-acting cardiotonic glyco-side to increase cardiac output, and aminophylline* to decrease bronchospasms and increase cardiac output.
Pulmonary embolism	• Emboli from thrombo-phlebitis • Venous stasis from pelvic trauma, obesity, varicose veins, preg-nancy, chronic heart fail-ure, MI, cancer, post-operative complications	• Dyspnea and tachypnea • Substernal pain, accompanied by apprehension and panic • Pallor or cyanosis • Fever, cough, hemoptysis • Neck vein distention • Pleural friction rub, accentuated pulmonic second sound, and gallop rhythm heard on auscultation • Abnormal ABG results: very low PO_2; normal or elevated PCO_2 • History of recent surgery	• Follow general guidelines listed earlier. • Give O_2 by facemask or nasal cannula. • Be prepared to intubate patient, if necessary. • Attach patient to cardiac monitor. • Draw arterial blood for blood gas measurements. • Get patient's prothrombin time. • Prepare patient for chest X-ray and lung scan. • Give analgesics and sedatives, as ordered. • Be prepared to give heparin I.V., to prolong clot-ting time, as ordered. *Important:* Before administer-ing heparin, know which other drugs your patient is taking. Also, have protamine sulfate* on hand to neutralize the heparin, if necessary.
Septic shock	• Bacterial infection (usually gram-negative)	• Cool, clammy skin; tachycardia; tachypnea; hypotension; increasing confusion; and diminished urine output • Low-grade fever of 100° to 101° F. (37.8° to 38.3° C.), except in burn patients who may be hypothermic • Metabolic acidosis, unless patient's hyperventilating, in which case he'd have respiratory alkalosis • Elevated WBC, BUN, and proteinuria • Gastrointestinal distress	• Follow general guidelines listed earlier. • Insert a Foley catheter, if ordered. • Draw an arterial blood sample to obtain blood gas measurements. • Connect patient to a cardiac monitor. • If ordered, assist doctor with insertion of arterial line for continuous blood pressure monitoring, also with insertion of Swan-Ganz catheter.

*Available in the United States and in Canada.

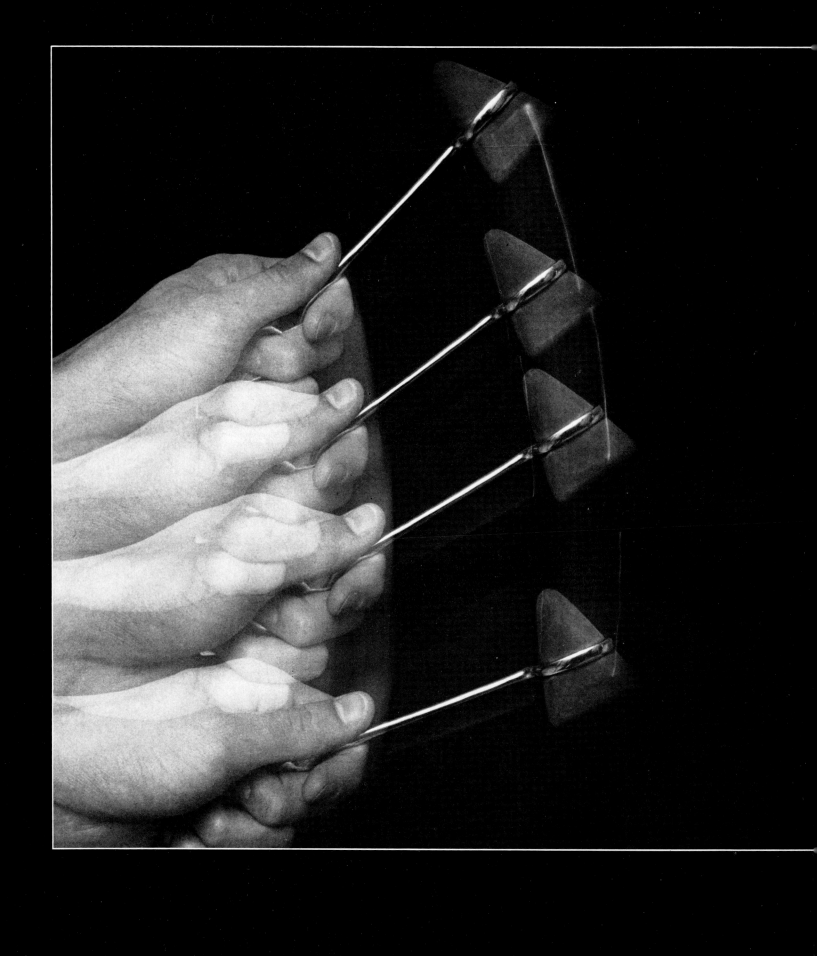

Managing Special Emergencies

Neurologic emergencies
Ob/Gyn guidelines
Neonatal emergencies

Neurologic emergencies

A neurologic emergency can be frightening to both you and your patient. So much depends on the quality of care the patient receives—and how quickly he receives it. For example, do you know what to do for a patient with a head injury? Your nursing skills may minimize the risk of dangerous complications and possibly save his life. Or in another case your know-how in moving a spinal-injury patient may prevent further neurologic damage.

Learn all you can about neurologic emergencies. Study the photostories, charts, and illustrations on these pages to find out how to properly assess and care for your patient. You never know when such information can help you save a patient's life.

Performing a neurologic assessment

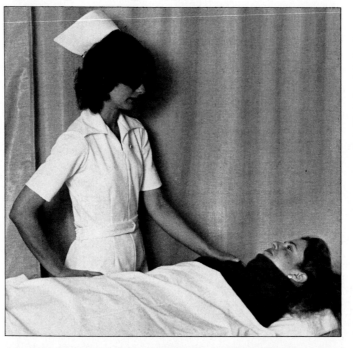

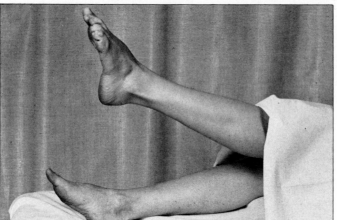

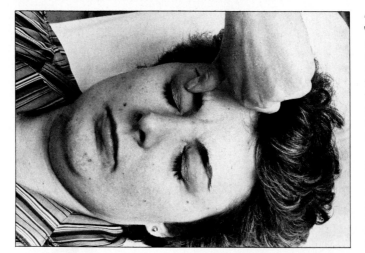

1 *When you perform the emergency assessment outlined on pages 10 to 13, you're checking your patient's level of consciousness and discovering whether she's oriented to time, place, and person. Asking these questions may seem silly to your patient, but they're important, because they help you assess the extent of her injuries.*

Suppose, for example, her answers suggest that she has a neurologic disorder caused by an injury to her head or spinal cord, or from some preexisting disease. Continue your neurologic assessment, using the guidelines in this photostory. (Remember, you already completed the first two steps in the neurologic evaluation process when you checked your patient's level of consciousness and her orientation.)

2 First, determine if your patient can respond to simple commands. Can she raise her leg, squeeze your hand, wiggle her toes? Ask her to perform several different acts, involving both sides of her body. Keep in mind that impaired motor function may account for her inability to respond.

3 Does she respond to pain? If your patient's unconscious, check by applying pressure to her nailbeds or the area over her eyes. Or, pinch the trapezius muscle ridge between her neck and shoulder. A patient with normal responses will try to withdraw from the stimulus or push it away.

Suppose your patient only grimaces or moves her body nonpurposefully. She may have a neurologic deficit. If she's paralyzed or comatose, she may not respond at all. Be specific when you make your observations.

4 Check your patient's corneal and gag reflexes. To test the corneal reflex, hold each eyelid open, and lightly stroke the cornea with the tip of a gauze pad. If she doesn't blink immediately, she may have a neurologic deficit and will need special eye care to prevent drying and irritation.

To test the patient's gag reflex, first depress her tongue with a wooden tongue depressor. Then, touch the back of her pharynx, on each side, with a cotton swab. If she doesn't gag, assume she'll need extra care, including suctioning, to prevent airway obstruction.

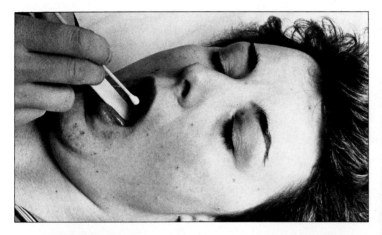

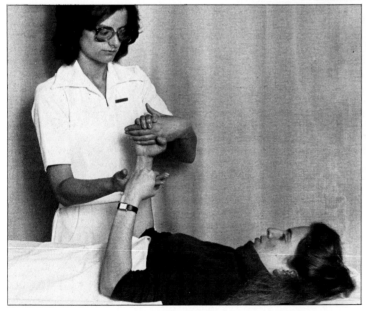

5 Test your patient's bilateral motor function. If you haven't already seen her move spontaneously, give her a simple command. For example, instruct her to squeeze both your hands simultaneously. Note if each handgrip is equal in strength.

Also check facial muscle movement. Can your patient smile? Close her eyes? Wrinkle her forehead? Watch closely for asymmetrical movement; for example, a drooping eyelid, drooping lip, or drooling.

If your patient exhibits an unusual movement, be sure to note it. Watch for spontaneous rigidity, rigidity in response to pain, reflex sucking and grasping, convulsive activity, and hiccuping.

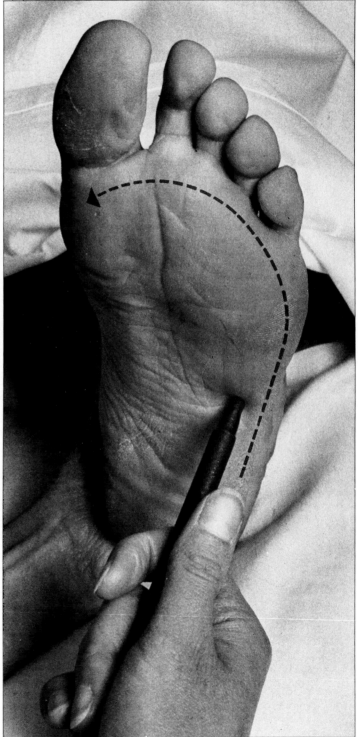

6 Check her plantar reflex by stroking the lateral aspect of her foot, on the sole, as shown here. If she flexes her toes downward, consider that a normal response. If she flexes her big toe up and her other toes out (the Babinski response), she may have a motor deficit.

Neurologic emergencies

Performing a neurologic assessment continued

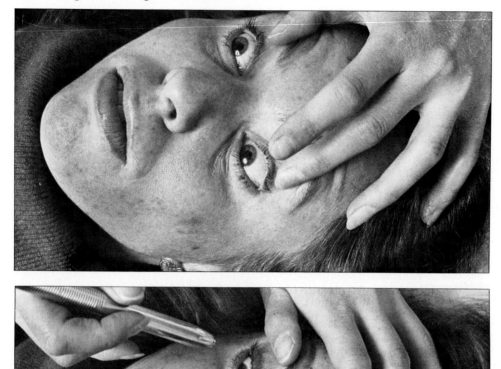

7 When you've completed these tests, check your patient's pupillary responses. (You already determined whether or not she had an eye prosthesis in your earlier assessment.) To check pupillary responses, hold the patient's eyelids open, and inspect her pupils for size, shape, and equality. Normally, pupils are round and of equal size, with a diameter ranging from 1.5 to 6 mm. However, your patient's pupil size may vary considerably from another patient's and still be considered normal. She may even have *unequal* pupils normally, which you may determine by asking her family the appropriate questions in your initial assessment. Be specific when you record your observations. Give pupil size in millimeters; don't use vague terms like "constricted" or "dilated."

8 Assess how your patient's pupils react to direct light. To do this, darken the room, and check each eye separately with a penlight. Moving from the side, shine the light directly into one pupil, as she keeps her other eye closed. If her pupil constricts properly with light, then dilates when the light is removed, consider this normal. If it doesn't, she may have a neurologic deficit.

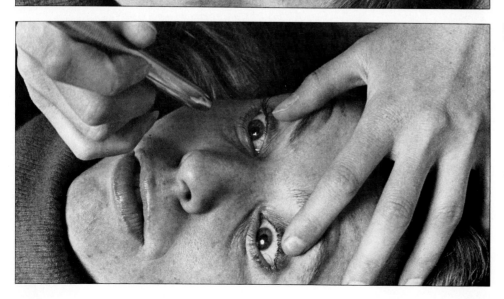

9 Also check the patient's pupils for consensual light reflex. To do so, hold both her eyelids open. Shine the light into one eye as you watch the other. Do the pupils constrict bilaterally? They should.

Document your findings when you've completed your assessment, and tell the doctor what you've observed. And remember, being specific with your information makes a difference. Your patient's life may depend on your efforts to report your evaluation accurately.

Nurses' guide to head and spinal cord emergencies

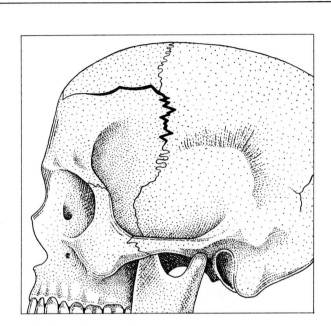

Problem
SKULL FRACTURE
(closed head injury; for example, simple concussion with brain tissue destruction, depressed skull fracture, or compound fracture of skull)

Causes
• Trauma

Signs and symptoms
• Loss of consciousness
• Coma, if patient has cerebral hemorrhage, contusion, or laceration of cortex
• Headache
• Nausea and vomiting
• Obvious deformity from skull depression

Emergency nursing considerations
• Watch for signs of increasing intracranial pressure and infection, and notify doctor.
• Don't administer sedatives, barbiturates, or morphine, as these may further depress your patient's respirations.
• If your patient has a simple concussion, keep him under close observation for 24 hours. If he's discharged, instruct his family to wake him every 2 hours the first night.
• Start I.V. therapy, if necessary, to keep patient hydrated, but restrict fluids administered to 1,500 to 2,000 ml daily.
• Keep accurate intake/output records.
• Monitor vital signs at least once every 2 hours.
• Draw arterial blood to obtain serial blood gas measurements to determine patient's respiratory status.
• Prepare patient for surgery, if ordered.
• Prepare to cleanse and suture any scalp lacerations. Use aseptic technique when caring for wounds to minimize risk of infection (a serious complication).
• Be prepared to assist doctor with immediate wound debridement and possible bone fragment removal. (Patient will require eventual surgery to correct skull fracture depression.)

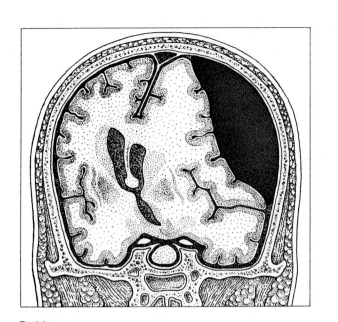

Problem
SUBDURAL HEMATOMA
(collection of blood between dura mater and arachnoid membrane)

Causes
• Head trauma; for example, from a fall or blow
• In newborn infant, may be caused by delivery complication

Signs and symptoms
• Headache
• Altered level of consciousness
• Hemiplegia on opposite side from hematoma
• Irritability, mental confusion
• Unequal pupils
• Convulsions
• Positive Babinski response
• Increased deep-tendon reflexes
• In infants: fever, hyperactive reflexes, bulging fontanelle, head enlargement, papilledema, paralysis, skull fracture

Emergency nursing considerations
• Make sure patient has open airway.
• Be ready to intubate patient, if necessary.
• Check patient's vital signs every 2 hours.
• Watch for signs of increasing intracranial pressure, and notify doctor.
• Obtain detailed history of trauma that caused hemorrhage.
• Intoxication may mask signs of this condition. Never forget that an intoxicated patient may also have a subdural hemorrhage.
• If the patient is a child or infant, consider the possibility of child abuse.

Neurologic emergencies

Nurses' guide to head and spinal cord emergencies continued

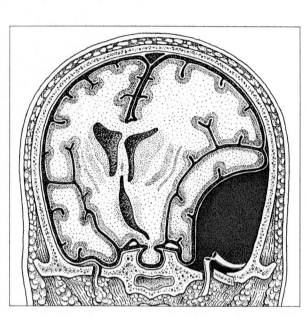

Problem
EXTRADURAL HEMORRHAGE: EPIDURAL HEMATOMA
(bleeding between skull and dura mater; the most life-threatening of intracranial hemorrhages because the bleeding is usually arterial)

Causes
- Trauma, causing tear in wall of middle meningeal artery
- Bleeding from dural sinus

Signs and symptoms
- Loss of consciousness, followed by a few hours of lucidity, then coma
- Hemiplegia on opposite side from hematoma
- Pupillary changes

Emergency nursing considerations
- Prepare patient for a computerized axial tomogram (CAT scan), if doctor orders. Remember, skull X-rays may show only linear fracture.
- If doctor orders, prepare patient for surgery.
- Watch for signs of increasing intracranial pressure, and notify doctor.
- Obtain detailed history of accident that caused hemorrhage.

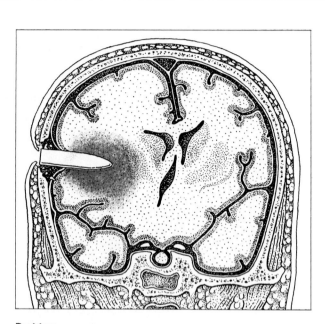

Problem
INTRACEREBRAL HEMORRHAGE
(sometimes widely dispersed)

Causes
- Fractured skull
- Penetrating skull injury
- Contracoup injury to skull
- Hemorrhagic disorders, such as aplastic anemia or leukemia

Signs and symptoms
- Headache
- Drowsiness
- Signs of increasing intracranial pressure
- Hemiplegia on opposite side from bleeding
- Dizziness
- Vomiting

Emergency nursing considerations
- Elevate patient's head to reduce venous pressure.
- Monitor his vital signs.
- Watch for signs of increasing intracranial pressure and notify doctor.
- Prepare patient for surgery, if ordered.

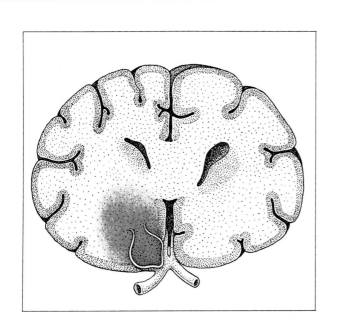

Problem
RUPTURED CEREBRAL ANEURYSM
(with subarachnoid hemorrhage)

Causes
- Congenital deformity of blood vessel wall
- Hypertension with atherosclerosis
- Trauma

Signs and symptoms
- Mild to severe headache
- Nuchal rigidity
- Hemiparesis or hemiplegia
- Ptosis
- Unilaterally dilated pupil
- Impaired vision from pressure on optic nerve
- Facial pain from pressure on fifth cranial nerve
- Dizziness
- Tinnitus

Emergency nursing considerations
- Closely monitor patient's vital signs, and watch for signs of increasing intracranial pressure.
- Put patient on complete bed rest, as ordered.
- Elevate patient's head to reduce venous pressure.
- Prepare patient for cerebral angiogram, if ordered.
- Prepare patient for lumbar puncture. (Doctor needs test to confirm diagnosis of blood in spinal fluid.)
- As ordered, give aspirin or codeine for headache.
- As ordered, give drugs to combat hypertension.
- Prepare patient for surgery, to clip aneurysm, if ordered.

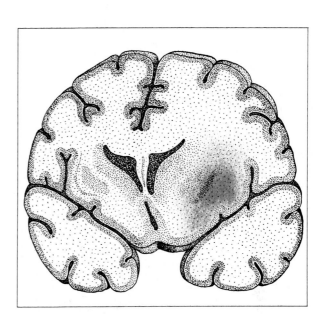

Problem
CEREBROVASCULAR ACCIDENT
(stroke)

Causes
- Thrombosis
- Embolus
- Hemorrhage

Signs and symptoms
- Sudden onset (on exertion) of signs and symptoms if stroke is caused by hemorrhage
- Slow, progressive onset of signs and symptoms if stroke is caused by thrombosis
- Acute onset of signs and symptoms if stroke is caused by embolus
- Partial to total paralysis; coordination loss
- Aphasia
- Headache
- Sensory impairment
- Incontinence
- Memory loss
- Visual disturbances
- Hypertension
- Convulsions
- Coma

Emergency nursing considerations
- Prepare patient for cerebral angiogram to determine aneurysm's location, if ordered.
- Make sure patient has open airway, and administer oxygen, as ordered.
- Closely monitor patient's vital signs, and watch for signs of increasing intracranial pressure.
- Do not administer morphine, because it may further depress your patient's respirations.
- Be alert for concurrent signs of myocardial infarction and atrial fibrillation.

Neurologic emergencies

Nurses' guide to head and spinal cord emergencies continued

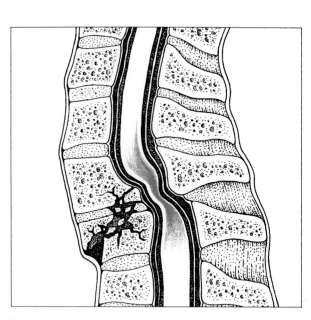

Problem
SPINAL CORD TRAUMA

Causes
• Penetrating injury
• Flexion or extension from fall, diving, or car accident
• In newborn infant, may be caused by traumatic (usually breech) delivery

Signs and symptoms
• Complete cord transection, resulting in permanent sensory or motor loss below injury level
• Incomplete transection, resulting in variable sensory and motor loss below injury level
• Spinal shock: rapidly decreasing blood pressure, decreased urinary output, and gastric distention

Emergency nursing considerations
• Immobilize patient immediately, using guidelines shown on page 140.
• Make sure the patient has an open airway, and be prepared to intubate him, if necessary.
• Control any external hemorrhaging.
• Prepare to transfer patient to CircOlectric bed, Stryker frame, or Rotorest frame, as ordered.
• If spinal shock occurs, start I.V. therapy with appropriate solution. Insert Foley catheter to relieve or prevent bladder distention. Insert nasogastric tube to relieve or prevent gastric distention.
• Do not give morphine because it will depress respirations.

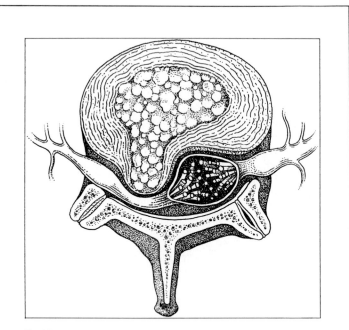

Problem
RUPTURED INTRAVERTEBRAL DISC

Causes
• Trauma

Signs and symptoms
• When trauma occurs in lumbar area, patient has pain in lower back, radiating down back of one leg. Also patient's paravertebral muscles are spastic, and his affected leg can't be straightened when his thigh is flexed.
• When trauma occurs in cervical area, patient has neck stiffness and local pain radiating down one arm to fingers.

Emergency nursing considerations
• Place patient in pelvic or cervical traction, if ordered.
• Prepare patient for myelogram, as ordered.
• Prepare patient for a laminectomy, if ordered.
• Give pain medication, as ordered.

Patient teaching

Your head injury: Some important reminders

Dear Patient:
Although you've suffered a head injury, the doctor doesn't feel that you have to be hospitalized at this time. He's found no evidence of serious injury.

However, for the next few days, you must watch your condition closely. If you develop *any* of the following signs and symptoms, call the doctor at once or come to the emergency department immediately:
- increasing drowsiness
- vomiting

- difficulty waking up. *Important:* During your first night at home, your family should awaken you every 2 hours.
- decreased pulse rate
- continual headache
- neck stiffness
- blood or clear fluid draining from ears or nose
- weakness in arms or legs; even one-sided weakness
- convulsions (fits).

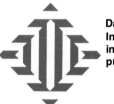

Danger: Increasing intracranial pressure

Your patient may show signs of increasing intracranial pressure (ICP) from any of the following conditions: intracranial hemorrhage, brain tumor, meningitis, or cerebral edema. Unless the condition is reversed, the patient's brain tissue will herniate through the tentorial notch, causing brain stem compression (see illustration at right).

To ensure prompt treatment, watch your patient closely for these danger signs:
- headache complaint (an early warning sign)
- decreasing level of consciousness
- vomiting
- change in pupil size or equality, papilledema, and extraocular movements. Remember, papilledema usually takes 12 to 24 hours to develop.
- rising blood pressure, slowing pulse, hyperthermia, and a change in respiration pattern (in later stage of ICP).

If you observe any of the above, notify the doctor at once. Document your findings in your nurses' notes.

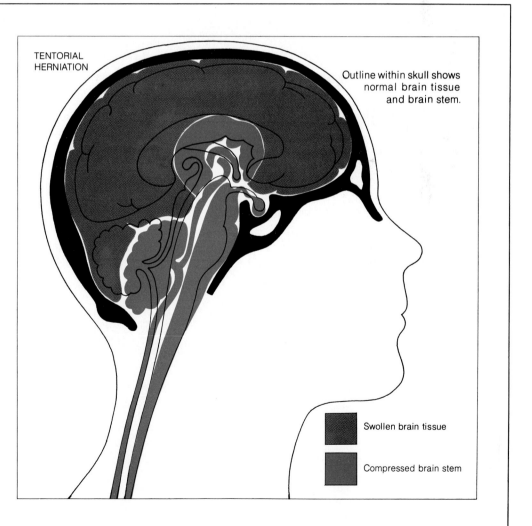

TENTORIAL HERNIATION

Outline within skull shows normal brain tissue and brain stem.

Swollen brain tissue

Compressed brain stem

Neurologic emergencies

How to cope with a seizure

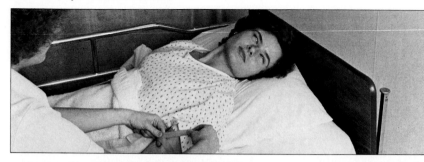

1 You're starting an I.V. on 22-year-old Cynthia Mc-
Fadden, who has a history of epilepsy. Suddenly,
she complains of "feeling strange," and based on your
previous experience with such patients, you suspect
she's about to have a seizure. Do you know what to do?
For example, what steps must you take to keep her
from hurting herself? What information should you
gather as you witness the seizure? What do you do
afterward? If you're not sure, read this photostory.

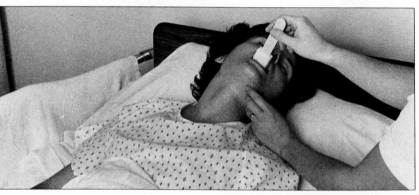

2 First, do your best to stay calm. If possible, place
a padded tongue depressor or disposable bite
block between your patient's teeth to keep her from bit-
ing her tongue. But don't attempt to force anything
between her teeth if they're already clenched; doing so
could cause injury. Work quickly. Call or signal for
help, but don't leave the patient. She could injure herself or choke to death while you're gone. Raise the side
rails on the bed, and pad them with a towel or bath
blanket.

Does the patient have dentures or an orthodontic
appliance? Try to remove these *before* you insert the
tongue depressor, but take care not to be bitten.

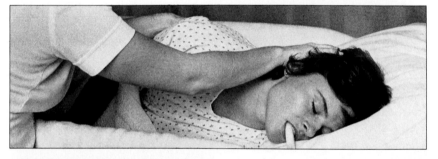

3 Position your patient on her side, with her head
back and her face slightly downward. This will
keep her airway open and permit saliva and vomitus to
drain from her mouth. (If you have a suctioning machine
nearby, you can use it to help clear secretions.)

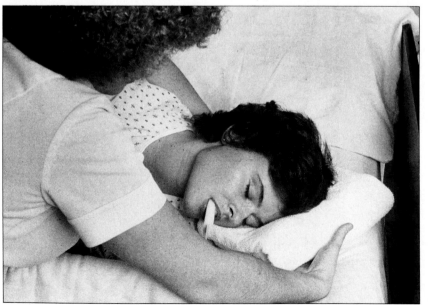

4 Place a small pillow or folded towel under your
patient's head as you position her. But take care
not to flex her neck so much you obstruct her airway.
Remove any extra pillows or bed linen that could get in
her way. Draw the bed curtain for privacy.

Never try to restrain your patient during the seizure. Doing so may make her convulsions more severe
and cause injury. In most cases, a seizure will last
only 2 to 5 minutes. Observe the patient closely during
this period to gather the information the doctor will
need later. (For details, see the box on the opposite
page.)

When the seizure is over, do your best to reassure
and reorient the patient. If she begins to have another
attack before regaining consciousness, consider the
possibility that she's developed status epilepticus,
which is a medical emergency.

In either case, notify the doctor immediately. Provide
him with the information you've gathered about the
seizure, and document your findings. Administer oxygen to the patient, if ordered by the doctor.

Transporting the patient with a spinal injury

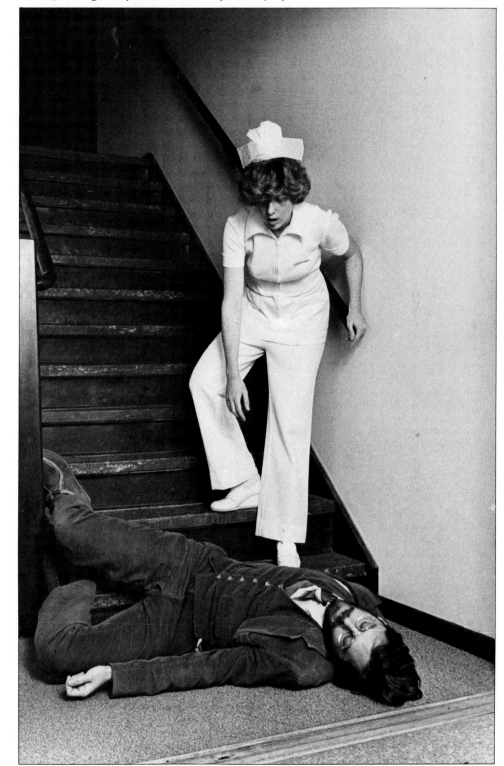

DOCUMENTING

Gathering seizure information

When you witness—and cope with—a patient's seizure, observe her carefully to collect the information needed by the doctor. Ask yourself the following questions, and do your best to remember what you saw.

• Exactly what time did the seizure occur?

• What was the patient doing just *before* the seizure, or what were you doing *to* her?

• How did the seizure develop? Gradually or suddenly? Did she complain of premonitory sensations? What part of her body started moving first? How did the convulsion spread?

• If your patient has been taking anticonvulsant drugs, when was her last dose?

• Did your patient change her position during the seizure?

• Did she chew, froth at the mouth, or roll her eyes?

• Were her eyes open throughout the seizure? If they were, what did her pupils look like? Did they dilate or constrict? Together or unilaterally?

• What were the patient's respirations like?

• What was the color and temperature of her skin?

• Was she incontinent?

• When did she regain consciousness? And how did she act then? Was she alert? Active? Or sleepy? Did she remember anything about the seizure or what preceded it? Did she have any injuries?

Document everything you remember in your nurses' notes. Notify the doctor of your findings.

1 *Let's assume you're on your way to the cafeteria when you see the hospital administrator, Jack Stephens, collapsed at the bottom of the stairway. Experience tells you he may have a spinal injury. So you immediately call for help. Would you know how to move him properly? If not, carefully follow the steps in this photostory.*

Neurologic emergencies

Transporting the patient with a spinal injury continued

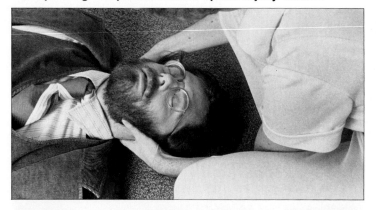

2 While you're waiting for help to arrive with a cervical collar, spine board, and stretcher, use your hands to immobilize Mr. Stephens' neck. To do this, gently grasp your patient's head, as the nurse is doing here, taking care to maintain his airway. Now, without applying pressure, cup your hands over your patient's ears. Place your fingers under his jaw, pointing toward each other. Using gentle traction, support your patient's head.

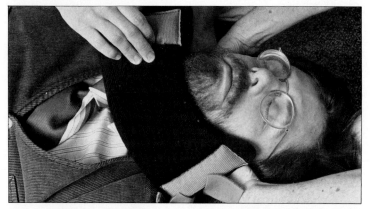

3 When help arrives, apply a cervical collar to Mr. Stephens' neck. To do so, continue to maintain manual traction while a coworker slips the collar in place. Then, release your hands. Make sure the collar fits snugly but not so tightly that it constricts his airway or circulation.
Nursing tip: If a commercially made cervical collar is not available, improvise one by rolling up a towel, sweater, or sheet, and place it around your patient's neck.

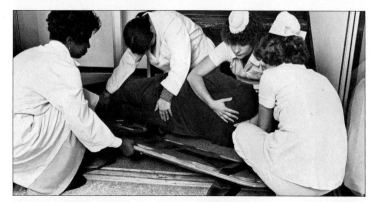

4 Before moving Mr. Stephens to a stretcher, you'll need to place him on the spine board. To get the spine board under your patient, have two coworkers turn him on his side, using a logrolling technique. Then, a third coworker slides the board into position, as shown here. Now, gently lower Mr. Stephens onto the board.

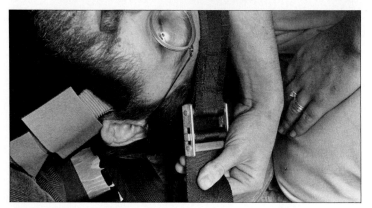

5 Firmly secure the straps at Mr. Stephens' head and chest. Next, using as much help as necessary, uniformly grip the spine board and lift it onto a stretcher, in one motion. Transport your patient to the ED for X-rays and diagnostic tests.

Transferring the patient with spinal injuries

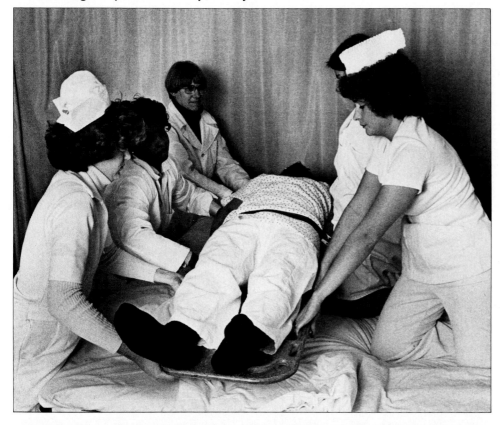

1 *As soon as Mr. Stephens arrives in the ED, he'll need immediate attention. Do you know how to help him?*

First, of course, do a quick emergency assessment, as explained on pages 8 and 9. Then, notify the doctor. Next, perform a more extensive neurologic assessment, as outlined on pages 130 to 132.

Make sure Mr. Stephens remains immobilized during all X-rays and diagnostic tests. To ensure this, always accompany your patient when he's transported for X-rays and testing. Never assume others will keep him immobilized.

Finally, prepare Mr. Stephens for surgery, if ordered by the doctor. Or, following doctor's orders, transfer him to another unit for treatment.

When the time comes to transfer Mr. Stephens from the stretcher to a bed, you'll need at least four coworkers to help you. Three coworkers should stand on one side of the stretcher and grip the spine board. Two other persons should position themselves on the opposite side of the bed, gripping the opposite edge of the board. On a predetermined signal, uniformly lift the spine board and move it onto the bed, as shown here. To remove your patient from the spine board, logroll him, making sure his spine stays perfectly aligned.

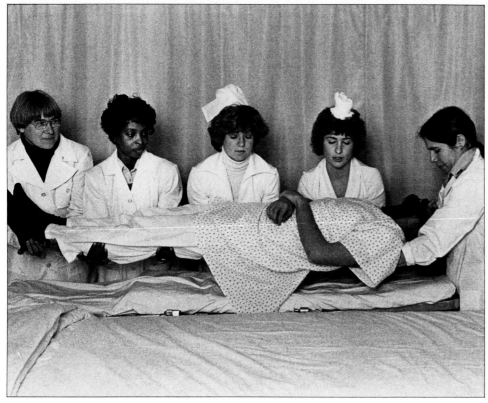

2 If your patient isn't on a spine board, use this method to transfer your patient from the stretcher to the bed. First, you'll need at least four coworkers to assist. Instruct three persons to stand on the same side of the stretcher, with their arms (palms up) under the patient. The leader—in most cases a doctor—stands at the patient's head to direct the transfer. She also supports the patient's head and neck. A fifth coworker stands at the patient's feet.

When the doctor says, "Lift," everyone must lift together, taking care to keep the patient's spine properly aligned, as shown in this photo. Once the patient's lifted, the person standing at his feet can move the stretcher safely out of the way. Then, slowly lower the patient onto the bed.

Neurologic emergencies

Providing spinal support for a diving accident victim

1 *Two hours after you finish your shift at the hospital, you're enjoying a relaxing swim in a health spa pool. Suddenly, you're aware that one of the other swimmers has had a diving accident. She needs immediate help. Do you know what to do?*

Assume she's suffered a spinal injury. As you swim toward her, shout for help, specifically requesting a firm support; for example, a spine board, surfboard, or door.

2 When you reach the victim and bring her to the surface, carefully roll her face up in the pool, as shown here. Using standard lifesaving technique, begin moving her toward the shallow end of the pool. As you do, keep her head and shoulders properly aligned. Assess her breathing, and administer artificial respiration, if needed.

3 As soon as help arrives, carefully slide the board under the victim while she's still in the water.

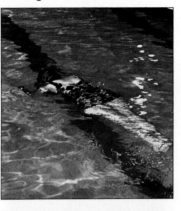

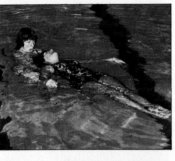

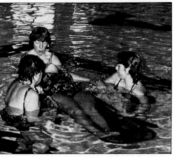

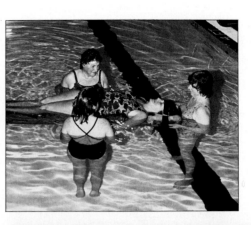

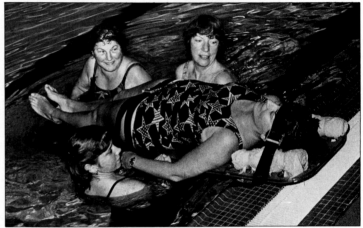

4 If you're using a regular spine board, buckle the headstrap over the patient's head. Further immobilize her by placing a rolled up towel on either side of her head and neck, as shown here.

5 Now, lift the victim from the pool, taking care not to alter her position on the spine board. If possible, apply a cervical collar to further immobilize her neck.

Continue to assess her breathing and administer artificial respiration (if needed) until an ambulance arrives. Give all relevant information about the accident to the emergency medical technicians.

TROUBLESHOOTING

When skull tongs slip out of place: What to do

Your newest patient is 17-year-old Jeff Martin, who fractured his neck at the C-5 level in a diving accident. As part of Jeff's treatment, the doctor immobilized his head and neck with skull tongs. Today, you discover that one of Jeff's tongs has slipped out of place. Obviously, you can't reinsert it, because that's the doctor's responsibility. What do you do?

First, call or signal for help. Then, carefully remove the traction weights to eliminate uneven tension on Jeff's head and spinal column. Next, immobilize his head and neck with 10- pound sandbags.

Nursing tip: Suppose no sandbags are available. Immobilize Jeff's head and neck with your hands. But don't be too forceful. Apply just enough pressure to keep his head and neck properly aligned.

Never leave a patient like Jeff alone. Ask the nurse who's come to your aid to get the doctor. Then, while you're waiting, check both tong insertion sites on Jeff's skull for a possible fluid leak. Such a leak, if it proves to be cerebrospinal fluid, will indicate that a tong has penetrated the patient's brain cavity.

When the doctor arrives, advise him of your findings and stand by, ready to assist. Then, document everything in your nurses' notes.

Another important reminder: Whenever you care for a patient with skull tongs, always keep two 10-pound sandbags at his bedside. Doing so will prepare you for this type of emergency.

Ob/Gyn guidelines

How familiar are you with gynecologic and obstetric emergencies? For example, do you know what to suspect—and do—if a young woman is rushed to the ED with severe pain in her left lower abdomen, vaginal bleeding, dizziness, and weakness? Or what if your patient's in her third trimester of pregnancy and suddenly develops hypertension, edema, and oliguria? Suppose you have to deliver a baby without a doctor's assistance. Can you do it?

On these pages, you'll learn how to recognize some of the more common gynecologic and obstetric emergencies—and how to cope with them. Study the step-by-step instructions we've provided. Be fully prepared the next time this type of emergency comes your way.

Nurses' guide to Ob/Gyn emergencies

Has it been awhile since you've cared for a patient with an Ob/Gyn emergency? If so, review the chart below.

Remember, in any Ob/Gyn emergency, you must monitor your patient closely for signs of shock and begin I.V. therapy, as needed, with the appropriate solution. Obtain a complete medical history from your patient, and reassure her and her family as much as possible. Explain all procedures clearly and calmly. Also, remember all Ob/Gyn emergencies require a high degree of empathy and understanding.

Problem
THREATENED ABORTION

Possible causes
- Reproductive tract trauma
- Reproductive tract abnormality or abnormality of developing fetus
- Acute infectious disease

Signs and symptoms
- Bright-red vaginal bleeding
- Mild cramps, although no cervical dilation is present
- Slight backache

Emergency nursing considerations
- Place patient in Trendelenburg position.
- Keep an accurate count of used perineal pads.
- Save any clots or tissue expelled by your patient, for examination by the doctor.
- Monitor your patient's vital signs closely.
- Draw blood for type, crossmatch, complete blood count (CBC), electrolyte determination, and Rh factor.
- If your patient's blood is Rh negative, give Rho (D) immune globulin* (RhoGam) I.M., as ordered by the doctor.
- If possible, move your patient to a quiet area to keep her from becoming more anxious.
- Prepare your patient for dilation and curettage (D & C), if ordered by doctor. *Caution:* No one should perform a rectal or vaginal examination on a patient with a threatened abortion.
- Avoid using the word abortion if your patient is more comfortable with the term miscarriage.

Problem
INEVITABLE, INCOMPLETE ABORTION

Possible causes
- Reproductive tract trauma
- Reproductive tract abnormality or abnormality of developing fetus
- Acute infectious disease

Signs and symptoms
- Conception products partially expelled, although the placenta may remain in the uterus
- Cervix dilated
- Profuse, bright-red vaginal bleeding
- Decreased blood pressure
- Increased pulse rate
- Gestation less than 20 weeks

Emergency nursing considerations
- Follow guidelines in introduction to chart.
- Follow the first five guidelines for threatened abortion.
- If your patient's blood is Rh negative, give Rho (D) immune globulin* (RhoGam) I.M., as ordered by the doctor.
- If possible, move your patient to a quiet area to keep her from becoming more anxious.
- Prepare your patient for dilation and curettage (D & C), if ordered by doctor. *Caution:* No one should perform a rectal or vaginal examination on a patient with a threatened abortion.
- Avoid using the word abortion if your patient is more comfortable with the term miscarriage.

Problem
COMPLETE ABORTION

Possible causes
- Reproductive tract trauma
- Reproductive tract abnormality or abnormality of developing fetus
- Endocrine disturbances
- Acute infectious disease

Signs and symptoms
- Complete expulsion of conception products
- Cervix dilated
- Moderate amount of vaginal bleeding

Emergency nursing considerations
- Follow guidelines in introduction to chart.
- Follow the first four guidelines for threatened abortion.
- Draw blood for type, crossmatch, complete blood count (CBC), electrolyte determination, and Rh factor.
- If your patient's blood is Rh negative, give Rho (D) immune globulin* (RhoGam) I.M., as ordered by the doctor.
- If possible, move your patient to a quiet area to keep her from becoming more anxious.
- Prepare your patient for dilation and curettage (D & C), if ordered by doctor. *Caution:* No one should perform a rectal or vaginal examination on a patient with a threatened abortion.
- Avoid using the word abortion if your patient·is more comfortable with the term miscarriage.
- Additionally, be ready to administer oxytocin (Pitocin* and Syntocinon*), as ordered by the doctor.

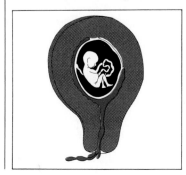

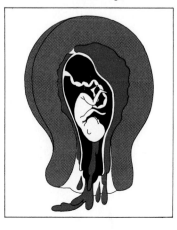

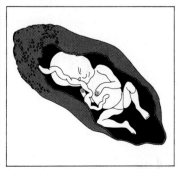

*Available in the United States and in Canada.

Ob/Gyn guidelines

Nurses' guide to Ob/Gyn emergencies continued

Problem
HABITUAL ABORTION
(woman aborts three or more times sequentially)

Possible causes
• Faulty intrauterine environment
• Cervical incompetence

Signs and symptoms
• Complete expulsion of conception products
• Cervix dilated
• Moderate amount of vaginal bleeding

Emergency nursing considerations
• Place patient in Trendelenburg position.
• Keep an accurate count of used perineal pads.
• Save any clots or tissue expelled by your patient, for examination by the doctor.
• Draw blood for type, crossmatch, complete blood count (CBC), electrolyte determination, and Rh factor.
• If your patient's blood is Rh negative, give Rho (D) immune globulin* (RhoGam) I.M., as ordered by the doctor.
• If possible, move your patient to a quiet area to keep her from becoming more anxious.
• Prepare your patient for dilation and curettage (D & C), if ordered by doctor. *Caution:* No one should perform a rectal or vaginal examination on a patient with a threatened abortion.
• Avoid using the word abortion if your patient is more comfortable with the term miscarriage.

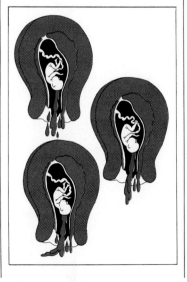

Problem
MISSED ABORTION
(fetal death, with conception products retained for several weeks or more)

Possible causes
• Reproductive tract abnormality or abnormality of developing fetus
• Acute infectious disease

Signs and symptoms
• Little, if any, vaginal bleeding
• Signs of infection, such as low-grade fever; pain or tenderness on examination or during sexual intercourse; and purulent, vaginal discharge
• Absent signs of fetal life (if previously present); for example, no heart tones, no movement

Emergency nursing considerations
• Place patient in Trendelenburg position.
• Keep an accurate count of used perineal pads.
• Save any clots or tissue expelled by your patient, for examination by the doctor.
• Draw blood for type, crossmatch, complete blood count (CBC), electrolyte determination, and Rh factor.
• If your patient's blood is Rh negative, give Rho (D) immune globulin* (RhoGam) I.M., as ordered by the doctor.
• If possible, move your patient to a quiet area to keep her from becoming more anxious.
• Prepare your patient for dilation and curettage (D & C), if ordered by doctor. *Caution:* No one should perform a rectal or vaginal examination on a patient with a threatened abortion.
• Avoid using the word abortion if your patient is more comfortable with the term miscarriage.

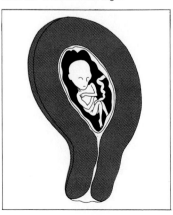

Problem
ECTOPIC PREGNANCY
(a pregnancy implanted outside the normal uterine cavity)

Possible causes
• Mechanical interference within fallopian tubes that prevents fertilized ovum from passing down toward the uterus; for example, developmental abnormalities of the tube or peritubal adhesions

Signs and symptoms
• If the fallopian tube's not ruptured, your patient will have amenorrhea, signs and symptoms of early pregnancy (for example, swollen breasts, morning sickness, frequent urination), dark-brown vaginal spotting, and adnexal discomfort
• If the fallopian tube's ruptured, your patient will have sudden sharp stabbing pain in her lower abdomen; shoulder-strap pain (Kehr's sign), and fixed abdominal tenderness when you turn her from side to side (Adler's sign).
• History of missed menstrual periods for 6 to 8 weeks before onset of pain
• Tenderness on vaginal exam, especially as cervix is moved
• Decreased blood pressure, proportional to blood loss
• Tender, boggy mass felt on one side of uterus
• Feeling of rectal pressure, accompanied by an urge to move bowels

Emergency nursing considerations
• Follow the first two guidelines from missed abortion.
• Prepare your patient for a pelvic examination by the doctor.
• Prepare your patient for culdocentesis, if ordered.
• Prepare your patient for surgery, if ordered; for example, a salpingectomy (with or without oophorectomy) or a laparoscopy.

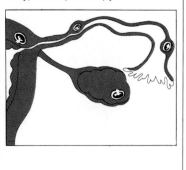

Problem
PLACENTA PREVIA
(implantation of any part of the placenta in the lower uterine segment)
Partial: internal os is partially covered by placenta
Total: internal os is totally covered by placenta
Marginal: part of placenta is attached to the lower uterine segment, with edge at the margin of cervical internal os

Possible causes
• Cause unknown

Signs and symptoms
• If patient is in her last trimester of pregnancy, she may have painless, vaginal bleeding that may gush intermittently or flow continuously.
• Placental souffle may be heard directly above the pubic symphisis with an ultrasonic Doppler

Emergency nursing considerations
• Place patient in semi-Fowler's position.
• Keep an accurate count of used perineal pads. Two saturated pads are equivalent to a pint of fluid loss.
• Be ready to attach a fetal monitor, as ordered by the doctor.
• Draw blood for type, crossmatch, complete blood count (CBC), platelets, fibrinogen index, prothrombin time (PT), partial thrombin time (PTT), chemistry profile.
• Prepare your patient for an emergency cesarean section, if ordered by the doctor.
• *Caution:* Don't give an enema or let anyone perform a vaginal or rectal examination on your patient; these may perforate the placenta.

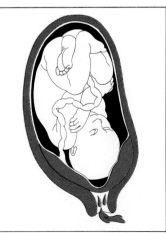

Problem
ABRUPTIO PLACENTAE
(complete or partial detachment of placenta from uterine wall, in third trimester)

Possible causes
- Cause unknown

Signs and symptoms
- With a marginal detachment of placenta, your patient will have vaginal bleeding. With a complete detachment of the placenta, your patient will have internal bleeding.
  Note: Bleeding that's internal collects in the myometrium, making the uterus tetanic, tender to the touch, and rigid (Couvelaire uterus). With severe bleeding, labor will cease. Your patient may show signs of shock, which may result in fetal death.
- Sudden, severe abdominal pain—knifelike at first, later becomes dull
- Backache
- Fetal heart sounds may be slow or absent (if fetus has died).
- Oliguria from shock, which can progress to acute renal failure

Emergency nursing considerations
- Monitor your patient's vital signs and the fetal heart rate.
- Draw blood for type, crossmatch, complete blood count (CBC), platelets, fibrinogen index, prothrombin time, partial thrombin time, and chemistry profile.
- Insert a Foley catheter, if ordered by the doctor. Monitor intake and output.
- Prepare your patient for Ultrasound B scan (to identify placenta and retroperitoneal clot).
- Prepare your patient and her family for an emergency cesarean section, if ordered by the doctor.
- Administer heparin and fibrinogen, as ordered by the doctor, to treat blood coagulation defects.

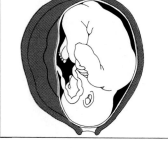

Problem
PROLAPSED UMBILICAL CORD
(umbilical cord is at or below the level of the presenting fetal part)

Possible causes
- Rupture of amniotic membrane, with presenting part of fetus above or not firmly against pelvic inlet. In most cases, the presenting part is a shoulder or foot.

Signs and symptoms
- Hydramnios (excessive fluid in amniotic sac)
- Umbilical cord seen on vaginal examination of your patient
- Fetal monitor may reflect irregular fetal heart rate, plus episodic spells of fetal hypoxia (shows as a dip on the monitor).

Emergency nursing considerations
- Call or signal for help immediately.
- Position your patient in knee-chest, or Trendelenburg position.
- Instruct your patient not to move.
- If umbilical cord's *inside* the vagina, insert your gloved hand, and elevate the presenting fetal part, to prevent cord compression.
- If the umbilical cord's *outside* the vagina, cover it with a sterile cloth soaked in warm normal saline solution. *Caution:* Don't try to replace the umbilical cord in the vagina.
- If your patient's completely dilated, prepare to assist the doctor with vaginal delivery. Otherwise, prepare your patient for an immediate cesarean section.

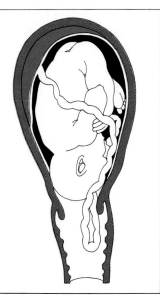

Problem
PRECLAMPSIA

Possible causes
- Cause unknown, but predisposing factors may include diabetes, chronic hypertension, multiple fetuses, or multiple sequential pregnancies.

Signs and symptoms
- Severe frontal headache
- Vision difficulties
- Repeated vomiting
- Oliguria
- Epigastric pain
- Hypertension
- Edema of face and hands
- Proteinuria

Emergency nursing considerations
- Carefully monitor your patient's vital signs and the fetal heart rate.
- Keep an emergency toxemia tray at your patient's bedside. This should include a padded tongue depressor (in case of convulsions) and all the drugs she may need, such as barbiturates, antihypertensives, sedatives, diuretics, and magnesium sulfate. Digitalis may be prescribed, if signs of cardiac failure are present.
- Record your patient's intake and output every hour, in case of renal shutdown.

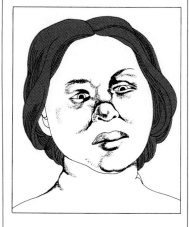

Problem
ECLAMPSIA

Possible causes
- Cause unknown, but predisposing factors may include diabetes, chronic hypertension, multiple fetuses, or multiple sequential pregnancies.

Signs and symptoms
- Severe frontal headache
- Vision difficulties
- Repeated vomiting
- Oliguria
- Epigastric pain
- Hypertension
- Edema of face and hands
- Proteinuria
- Convulsions

Emergency nursing considerations
- Follow guidelines listed for preclampsia.
- If your patient is convulsing, place her on a flat surface, with a folded handkerchief or padded tongue depressor between her teeth. However, never try to force a tongue depressor in your patient's mouth if her teeth are already clenched.
- Pad the side rails of the stretcher or bed. Wipe away any oral secretions, and turn her head to one side to prevent aspiration of vomitus. *Caution:* Never restrain your patient or leave her alone.

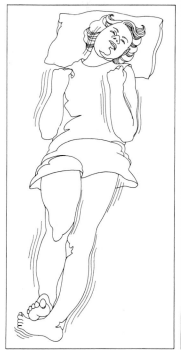
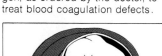

Ob/Gyn guidelines

Nurses' guide to Ob/Gyn emergencies continued

Problem
POSTPARTUM HEMORRHAGE
(blood loss of more than 500 ml, following birth of infant)

Possible causes
- Uterine atony
- Lacerations of reproductive tract
- Retained placental tissue

Signs and symptoms
- Steady blood flow from vagina
- When bleeding occurs after placental delivery and the fundus feels firm, suspect lacerations.
- On abdominal palpation, uterus may feel large and boggy.
- When pressure is applied to the uterus, patient expels large amounts of blood clots and fresh blood.
- Hypovolemic shock (for example, weak, rapid pulse; rapid, shallow respirations; low blood pressure; pallor; cold perspirations; dizziness; faintness; restlessness; and irritability)

Emergency nursing considerations
- Follow guidelines listed in introduction to chart.
- Stay with your patient, and massage the fundus while someone else notifies the doctor.
- Place your patient in the Trendelenburg position.
- If bleeding is caused by a retained placenta, prepare to help the doctor remove it.
- If the bleeding is caused by lacerations, prepare to help the doctor apply sutures. (In some cases, the patient may require surgical repair in the operating room.)
- Administer oxytocin as ordered by the doctor.

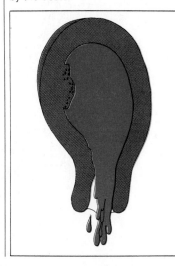

Problem
UTERINE RUPTURE

Possible causes
- Trauma from knife wound or auto accident
- Previous uterine scar
- Previous operative scar

Signs and symptoms
- Sudden acute abdominal pain during a contraction
- On abdominal palpation, you feel a contracted uterus and a hard mass alongside fetus
- Abdominal tenderness
- With a complete rupture, look for signs of internal bleeding.
- Contractions will cease.

Emergency nursing considerations
- Follow guidelines listed in introduction to chart.
- If the doctor determines the rupture is caused by a laceration, prepare to help the doctor apply sutures.
- Prepare your patient for a laparotomy and a hysterectomy, if ordered by the doctor.
- Administer antibiotics to prevent infection.

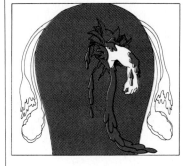

Problem
AMNIOTIC FLUID, OR MECONIUM EMBOLISM
(amniotic fluid or meconium enters venous sinuses of placental site and is drawn into the circulatory system, eventually reaching pulmonary capillaries)

Possible causes
- Anaphylactoid shock from presence of amniotic fluid or meconium in pulmonary arterioles

Signs and symptoms
- Sudden dyspnea
- Cyanosis
- Pulmonary edema
- Uterine relaxation
- Postpartum hemorrhage

Emergency nursing considerations
- Follow guidelines listed in introduction of chart.
- Notify the doctor immediately, as death may result a few minutes after symptoms appear.
- Administer oxygen, as needed.
- Be prepared to provide respiratory support.
- Closely monitor your patient's vital signs, central venous pressure, and urine output.

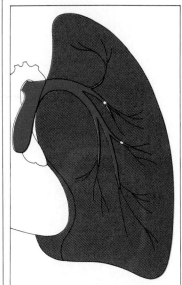

Problem
PULMONARY EMBOLISM

Possible causes
- A blocked pulmonary artery from detached thrombus. May be caused by a uterine or pelvic examination, or as a complication of delivery.

Signs and symptoms
- Sudden, intense dyspnea
- Patient unable to catch her breath

Emergency nursing considerations
- Follow guidelines listed in introduction to chart.
- Notify the doctor immediately.
- Administer high concentrations of oxygen by nasal cannula, followed by a mask or tent, as ordered by the doctor.
- Administer morphine and heparin, as ordered by the doctor.
- Be prepared to provide respiratory support.
- Monitor your patient's vital signs closely.

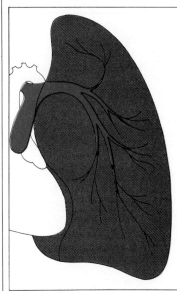

Ob/Gyn guidelines

How to deliver an infant

1 *Imagine this situation: You're almost ready to leave the hospital for the night when ambulance attendants bring in Rita Keller, a pregnant 34-year-old accountant. They tell you Mrs. Keller's pregnancy is full term (40 weeks) and she's in the transitional stage of labor.*

Since your hospital doesn't have an Ob/Gyn unit, you'll have to prepare for an emergency delivery. Here's what to do:

First, gather the equipment you'll need: large sterile basin (for the placenta), scissors, two medium Kelly clamps, bulb aspirator, umbilical cord tie, sterile gauze pads, sterile towels, plastic sheeting, blankets, and sterile mask and gloves.

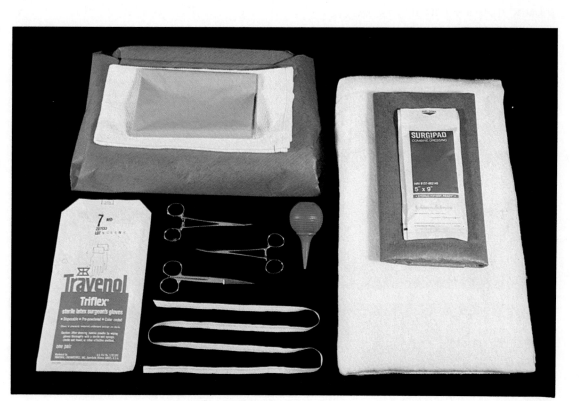

2 Now, make Mrs. Keller as comfortable as possible. Place her on her back, with her legs bent and her hands supporting her thighs, as shown here. Instruct a coworker to monitor Mrs. Keller's vital signs and the fetal heart rate. Offer support and encouragement. Explain to Mrs. Keller what you're going to do and how she can help. Encourage her to pant during her contractions to allow for a slow, gentle delivery.

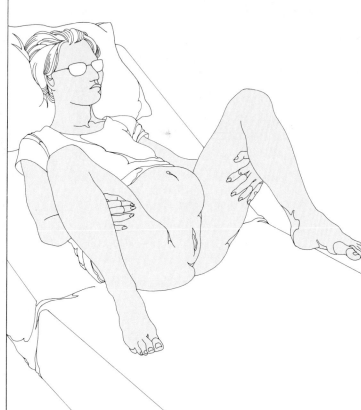

3 If time permits, wash Mrs. Keller's perineum with soap and water or surgical disinfectant. Put on sterile gloves and mask. Position the sterile basin on the bed, as close as possible to the vaginal opening. Place plastic sheeting under your patient's hips, and extend the lower edge into the basin. Cover the plastic with sterile towels.

Ob/Gyn guidelines

How to deliver an infant continued

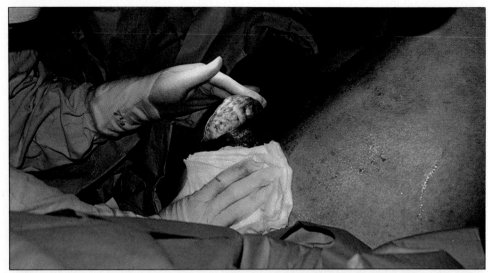

4 As the infant's head begins to crown, use the palm of your hand to apply gentle pressure to his head and to your patient's perineal area. *Caution:* Never exert *forceful* pressure on the infant's head. If you have time, use your other hand to position a gauze pad between Mrs. Keller's vaginal opening and the crowning head to protect it from the anus.

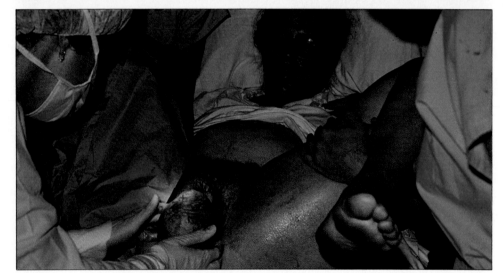

5 Now, carefully support the infant's head with both hands as it emerges from the vagina, as shown in this photo. Allow his head to rotate to one side.

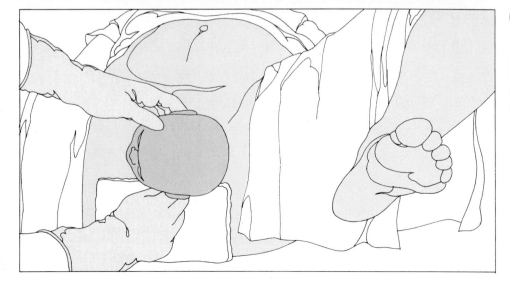

6 Now, slip your finger around the infant's neck, and feel for the umbilical cord. If it's loosely wrapped around his neck, you may be able to slip the cord over his head. If it's wrapped too tightly for that, clamp the cord in two places. Then, using sterile equipment, carefully cut between the clamps.

7 As you support the infant's head with one hand, wipe any mucus from his face, with gauze. Remove any remnants of the amniotic sac from the infant's face by carefully snipping them at the base of his neck. Then, quickly pull these remnants away from his face and airway. Suction the infant's nose and mouth with a bulb aspirator, to open his airway.

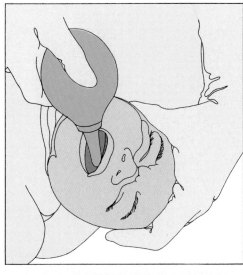

8 Next, begin to deliver the infant's shoulders. Instruct Mrs. Keller to bear down during the next contraction. Position your hands on either side of the infant's head, remembering to support his neck. Exert gentle downward pressure as you deliver his anterior shoulder.

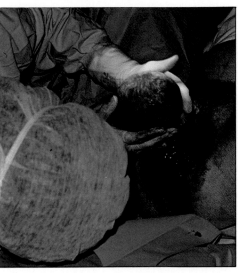

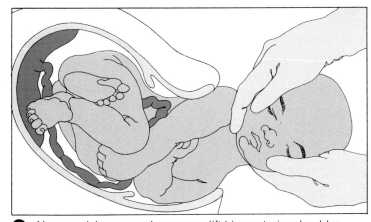

9 Now, applying upward pressure, lift his posterior shoulder. Support the rest of the infant's body as he's completely delivered. *Caution:* Don't force the infant upward. Undue pressure may damage spinal cord nerves in his neck.

10 Use the full length of your arm to firmly support the infant, as shown here. Keep him at a level below or equal to his mother until the umbilical cord stops pulsating.
   Caution: Never suspend an infant by his feet. If he doesn't cry spontaneously, gently rub or pat his back or the soles of his feet.

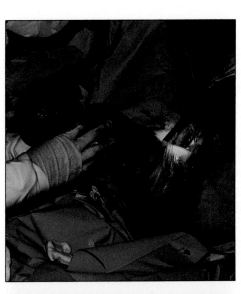

11 When the umbilical cord stops pulsating, use the Kelly clamps to clamp it. Position the clamps 1″ to 2″ (2.5 to 5 cm) apart. Once you've clamped the cord, don't be in a rush to cut it. Instead, place the infant on Mrs. Keller's abdomen, and cover him with a warm blanket, as shown here.

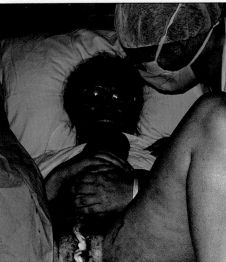

12 If you have sterile equipment, cut cord between the clamps and tie it in two places, about 3″ (7.6 cm) from infant's abdomen. Usually, tying the cord 1½″ to 2″ (3.8 to 5 cm) from infant's abdomen would be enough, but since there may be a blood incompatibility, leave 3″ (7.6 cm), so a blood exchange can be performed, if needed.

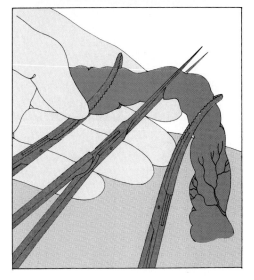

Ob/Gyn guidelines

How to deliver an infant continued

13 Have your coworker maintain the infant's open airway. At the same time, she'll assess his Apgar rating at 1 minute after birth and again at 5 minutes. (For more details on the Apgar scoring system, see page 153.) Place him on his side with Mrs. Keller or in the Isolette, in clear view. If the infant's cord stump begins bleeding at any time, notify the doctor.

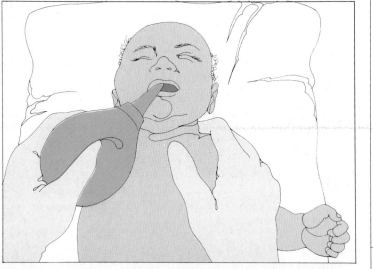

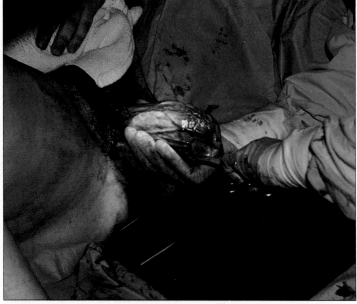

14 Within 5 minutes after the infant's been delivered, the placenta should separate from the uterine wall. Stay alert for separation signs, such as dark blood gushing from the vagina, lengthening of umbilical cord, uterine fundus rising upward in the patient's abdomen, or her uterus becoming firmer. When you see these signs, placental separation has begun. Encourage Mrs. Keller to bear down, to expel the placenta. Then apply gentle downward pressure on the abdomen to aid placental delivery. Make sure that you save the placenta in the basin so the doctor can inspect it. Check for evidence of retained placenta, which may cause maternal hemorrhage.

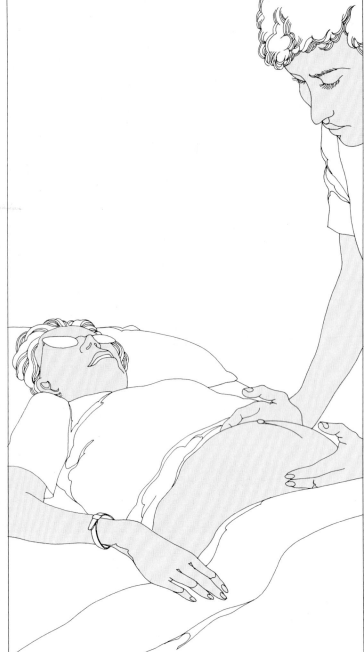

15 Continue to observe Mrs. Keller for vaginal bleeding and shock. Notify the doctor, if necessary. Check her uterine fundus every 15 minutes. Massage it as soon as it shows signs of relaxing. Also, check the patient's vaginal and perineal area for excessive bleeding. Have oxytocin (Pitocin*, Syntocinon*) available to stimulate myometrial contractions. Watch for lacerations of the vagina, and have suture material available.

Keep the mother and infant warm. Place an identification band on each, and prepare them for transfer. Also, prepare to transfer them to another unit. Finally, document the procedure in your nurses' notes.

*Available in the United States and in Canada.

Neonatal emergencies

Nurses' guide to neonatal emergencies

Coping with neonatal emergencies can be difficult if you're not sure what to look for. Remember, your ability to make quick, accurate patient observations may prevent a full-fledged crisis. We've provided the chart below to familiarize you with the most common neonatal emergencies.

Problem
PREMATURITY

Possible causes
• Multiple birth
• Eclampsia
• Maternal trauma
• Toxemia
• Antepartum hemorrhage
• Rh incompatibility
• Maternal history of cardiac disease, diabetes, chronic malnutrition, or severe infection
• History of premature births
• Habitual abortions

Signs and symptoms
• Respiratory distress (as described earlier)
• Small-sized infant, with thin, wrinkled skin, and limpness
• Excessive lanugo
• Relatively large head
• Protruding abdomen
• Absent or diminished sucking, swallowing, and gag reflexes

Emergency nursing considerations
• Place infant in an Isolette to keep him warm and to prevent possible infections.
• Monitor infant's respirations. If he shows signs of distress, place him on apnea and cardiac monitors, and administer oxygen.
• Prepare to assist the doctor with a tracheotomy, if ordered.
• Administer medications, as ordered by the doctor.

Problem
IMPERFORATE ANUS

Possible causes
• Congenital abnormality

Signs and symptoms
• On examination, no anal opening is found
• Absence of meconium stool
• Attempt to insert a small finger or thermometer into the infant's rectum is unsuccessful
• Developing abdominal distention

Emergency nursing considerations
• Prepare the infant for gastric suction, until surgery is scheduled.
• If the distance from infant's anus to intestine is greater than ½" (1.3 cm), the doctor may want to perform a colostomy. Prepare infant for surgery, if necessary.
• If a colostomy is performed, provide good skin care around colostomy site.

Problem
HYALINE MEMBRANE DISEASE

Possible causes
• Premature birth
• Complication of cesarean delivery

Signs and symptoms
• Respiratory distress; for example, nasal flaring, pallor, cyanosis, xiphoid retractions, atonia or hypotonia, respiratory grunts, and respiratory rate over 60 per minute
• Feeble cry
• Poor or absent sucking reflex

Emergency nursing considerations
• Place infant in Isolette, as ordered.
• Monitor infant's vital signs closely. Administer oxygen, if necessary, and be prepared to place him on an apnea monitor.
• Draw arterial blood for blood gas measurements, as ordered by the doctor.
• Administer medications, as ordered by the doctor.
• Be ready to place infant on mechanical ventilation, if necessary.

Problem
HYPERBILIRUBINEMIA

Possible causes
• Rh incompatibility
• ABO incompatibility
• Prematurity
• Sepsis
• Drugs
• Enlarged liver or spleen
• Dark yellow or straw-colored amniotic fluid at birth
• Jaundiced skin and mucous membranes

Signs and symptoms
• In kernicterus or bilirubin encephalopathy, infant has spasticity, reflex loss, high-pitched cry, lethargy, developing rigidity, hypotonia, opisthotonos (with or without seizures).

Emergency nursing considerations
• Check mother's blood type. If she's Rh negative, also check father's blood type. Get a complete history of her pregnancy and labor.
• Prepare for a blood transfusion. (For details, see the NURSING PHOTOBOOK *Managing I.V. Therapy.*)
• If phototherapy is ordered, check the lamp's age. If it's been used over 200 hours, it may be ineffective. Warm room before you remove the infant's clothing. Be sure his eyes are covered with eye patches or a bilimask.
• Administer I.V. fluids or oral feedings, as ordered, to keep infant well hydrated.
• Monitor fluid intake closely.
• Monitor infant's vital signs closely.
• Draw blood and collect urine sample for bilirubin test, as ordered by the doctor.
• Be prepared to give anticonvulsant drugs, as ordered by the doctor, to help control or prevent seizures.

Neonatal emergencies

Nurses' guide to neonatal emergencies continued

Problem
INTRACRANIAL HEMORRHAGE

Possible causes
* Trauma at birth; for example, hard or precipitous labor and delivery, forceps injury
* Hypoxia from placenta previa, abruptio placentae, hypotension, umbilical cord pressure, or precipitous or hard labor and delivery

Signs and symptoms
* Vomiting
* Lethargy
* Poor sucking reflex
* Irregular, difficult respirations, cyanosis
* Pale, cool clammy skin
* Anxious expression
* High-pitched cry
* Several hours following birth, twitching or generalized convulsions
* Within 12 to 24 hours, baby progresses from flaccidity to spasticity
* Unequal pupils
* Tense or bulging fontanelle, skull distortion
* Nuchal rigidity

Emergency nursing considerations
* Move infant to quiet, warm environment.
* Assist doctor with a diagnostic spinal tap, if ordered.
* Be prepared to assist with subdural tap, as ordered.
* Administer oxygen, if respiratory distress occurs.
* Slightly elevate infant's head.
* Administer I.V. fluids to keep infant well hydrated, as ordered by the doctor.

Problem
DRUG WITHDRAWAL

Possible causes
* Drug-addicted mother

Signs and symptoms
* Irritability, hyperactivity, tremors
* Vomiting
* Uncoordinated sucking and swallowing
* Shrill, high-pitched cry
* Resists cuddling

Emergency nursing considerations
* Place infant on his side; support his back with a small pillow or towel. Turn him every hour.
* Dim the lights, and decrease the noise level, if possible.
* Give small (30 ml) feedings every 30 to 60 minutes (depending on individual responses) to reduce vomiting.
* Monitor infant's vital signs closely.
* Place infant on apnea monitor. Watch for seizures. If seizures develop and apnea occurs, flick his feet to stimulate breathing.
* Be prepared to give infant phenobarbital, paregoric, chlorpromazine, or diazepam to wean him from heroin.
* Swaddle and hold infant to soothe him.
* If possible, get a complete medical history from the mother, including all drugs she's taken.

Problem
ESOPHAGEAL ATRESIA

Possible causes
* Esophageal abnormality. (Suspect this condition when mother has polyhydramnios.)

Signs and symptoms
* Cyanosis, as secretions accumulate
* During feedings, choking and excessive salivation

Emergency nursing considerations
* Discontinue oral feedings until infant is further evaluated.
* Place infant on his side, and keep his head elevated.
* Administer oxygen and I.V. fluids, as ordered.
* Suction pharyngeal airway frequently to prevent aspiration of mucus.
* Prepare infant for whatever immediate surgical intervention the doctor orders; for example, a tracheotomy, chest tubes, or gastrostomy. Eventually, however, the infant will require complete surgical correction of the condition.

Problem
MENINGOCELE

Possible causes
* Congenital malformation of spinal cord; i.e., spina bifida

Signs and symptoms
* Large globular sac protruding from base of infant's spinal column. Sac contains meninges and cerebrospinal fluid, and is translucent against direct light.
* Hydrocephalus (not always evident immediately). Early signs include tense fontanelle and increased head size.

Emergency nursing considerations
* Position infant correctly, according to doctor's orders, and check him hourly. In most cases, elevate the infant's head slightly, then place him either on his abdomen, with his feet hanging over the mattress edge, or on his side. Immoblize him with sandbags or blanket rolls, if necessary, to keep him from rolling onto his back. The doctor may also want you to use a Bradford frame, to allow urine and feces to drain from the infant's body.
* Prevent fecal and urinary contamination of sac by keeping infant's buttocks and genitalia clean. Place a disposable pad under the infant instead of diapering him. Tape a small plastic drape between sac and anus.
* To keep the sac from becoming irritated or ruptured, apply warm, moist compresses, as ordered. Be prepared to administer an antibiotic drip to sac's surface to prevent infection.
* Monitor the infant's vital signs closely.
* Administer I.V. fluids, as ordered by the doctor.
* Stay alert for signs of infection by watching the infant closely and taking his axillary temperature hourly. Notify the doctor immediately if the infant develops fever or has drainage from sac, concentrated or foul-smelling urine, opisthotonos, or convulsions.
* If necessary, be prepared to assist the doctor with insertion of a nasogastric tube.
* Prepare infant for surgery. Chances are, the doctor will schedule it within 24 hours after the infant's birth.
* Explain all procedures to infant's parents.

Problem
MENINGOMYELOCELE

Possible causes
● Congenital malformation of spinal cord; for example, spina bifida

Signs and symptoms
● Large globular sac protruding from base of infant's spinal column. Sac contains portion of spinal cord, meninges, and cerebrospinal fluid. Bluish area near sac's top indicates exposed neural tissue.
● Clubbed feet
● Loss of motor control and sensation below sac
● Increases susceptibility to meningitis and contractures in ankles, hips, and knees
● Impaired bowel and bladder function

Emergency nursing considerations
● Follow the guidelines listed for meningocele.
● Check for bladder distention. Credé bladder, if needed.
● Observe for signs of infection, hydrocephalus, or nerve damage, such as increasing weakness, paralysis, lethargy, listlessness, vomiting, and convulsions.

Problem
INTESTINAL OBSTRUCTION

Possible causes
● Congenital atresia or intestinal stenosis
● Malrotation of the colon with volvulus
● Meconium ileus
● Internal hernias
● Hirschsprung's disease

Signs and symptoms
● Abdominal distention
● Absence of stools
● Bile-stained vomitus

Emergency nursing considerations
● Place infant in semi-Fowler's position to ease respirations.
● Discontinue oral feedings until infant is further evaluated.
● Administer I.V. fluids, as ordered by the doctor, to keep infant well hydrated.
● Prepare to assist doctor with insertion of a nasogastric tube for gastric decompression. Attach the nasogastric tube to the low intermittent suction, if ordered.
● Prepare infant for surgery, if ordered by the doctor.

MINI-ASSESSMENT

Using the Apgar scoring system
To help assess a newborn infant's condition, check him against the Apgar scoring system shown here. Study the chart carefully; then make your observations within 1 minute after the infant's delivered; then again within 5 minutes.

Notify the doctor of your findings, and document them on the infant's chart. As a rule, you can consider a newborn infant vigorous if his rating totals 7 or above.

Apgar scoring system (select appropriate rating)

Sign	0	1	2	Rating 1 min.	Rating 5 min.
Heart rate	Not detectable	Slow (below 100)	Over 100		
Respiratory effort	Absent	Slow, irregular	Good, crying		
Muscle tone	Flaccid	Some flexion of extremities	Active motion		
Reflex irritability 1. Response to slap on sole of foot or	No response	Grimace	Cry		
2. Response to catheter in nostril (tested after oropharynx is clear)	No response	Grimace	Cough or sneeze		
Color	Blue, pale	Body pink, extremities blue	Completely pink		
Scoring system developed by Dr. Virginia Apgar			FINAL TOTAL		

Selected references

Books

American National Red Cross. BASIC FIRST AID. Garden City, N.Y.: Doubleday & Co., 1977.

Artz, Curtis P., et al. BURNS: A TEAM APPROACH. Philadelphia: W.B. Saunders Co., 1979.

Artz, Curtis P., et al. THE TREATMENT OF BURNS. Philadelphia: W.B. Saunders Co., 1969.

Barry, J. EMERGENCY NURSING. New York: McGraw-Hill Book Co., 1977.

Bergersen, Betty S. PHARMACOLOGY IN NURSING, 14th ed. St. Louis: C.V. Mosby Co., 1979.

Bolognese, Ronald, and Richard H. Schwarz, eds. PERINATAL MEDICINE: CLINICAL MANAGEMENT OF THE HIGH RISK FETUS AND NEONATE. Baltimore: Williams & Wilkins Co., 1977.

Brunner, Lillian S., and Dorothy S. Suddarth. THE LIPPINCOTT MANUAL OF NURSING PRACTICE, 2nd ed. Philadelphia: J.B. Lippincott Co., 1978.

Brunner, Lillian S., et al. TEXTBOOK OF MEDICAL-SURGICAL NURSING, 4th ed. Philadelphia: J.B. Lippincott Co., 1980.

Chung, Edward K., ed. CARDIAC EMERGENCY CARE. Philadelphia: Lea & Febiger, 1975.

Clark, Ann L., et al. CHILDBEARING: A NURSING PERSPECTIVE, 2nd ed. Philadelphia: F.A. Davis Co., 1979.

Clausen, Joy, et al. MATERNITY NURSING TODAY, 2nd ed. New York: McGraw-Hill Book Co., 1977.

Cosgriff, James H., Jr., and Diann Anderson. THE PRACTICE OF EMERGENCY NURSING. Philadelphia; J.B. Lippincott Co., 1975.

Dickason, Jean, and Martha Schult. MATERNAL AND INFANT CARE, 2nd ed. New York: McGraw-Hill Book Co., 1979.

Feller, I., and C. Archambeault-Jones. NURSING THE BURNED PATIENT. Ann Arbor, Mich.: National Institute for Burn Medicine, 1973.

GIVING CARDIOVASCULAR DRUGS SAFELY. Nursing Skillbook® Series. Springhouse, Pa.: Intermed Communications, Inc., 1978.

GIVING EMERGENCY CARE COMPETENTLY. Nursing Skillbook® Series. Springhouse, Pa.: Intermed Communications, Inc., 1978.

Hudak, Carolyn M., et al. CRITICAL CARE NURSING, 2nd ed. Philadelphia: J.B. Lippincott Co., 1977.

Jensen, Margaret, et al. MATERNITY CASE: THE NURSE AND THE FAMILY. St. Louis: C.V. Mosby Co., 1977.

Kintzel, Kay C., et al. ADVANCED CONCEPTS IN CLINICAL NURSING, 2nd ed. Philadelphia: J.B. Lippincott Co., 1977.

Loebl, Suzanne, et al. THE NURSE'S DRUG HANDBOOK. New York: John Wiley & Sons, Inc., 1977.

McSwain, M.E., ed. TRAUMATIC SURGERY. New York: Medical Examination Publishing Co., Inc., 1976.

MANAGING I.V. THERAPY. Nursing Photobook™ Series. Springhouse, Pa.: Intermed Communications, Inc., 1980.

Marlow, Dorothy R. A TEXTBOOK OF PEDIATRIC NURSING, 5th ed. Philadelphia: W.B. Saunders Co., 1977.

Meltzer, L.E., et al. CONCEPTS AND PRACTICES OF INTENSIVE CARE FOR NURSE SPECIALISTS. Bowie, Md.: Charles Press Publishers, 1976.

Mereness, Dorothy A., and Cecilia M. Taylor. ESSENTIALS OF PSYCHIATRIC NURSING, 10th ed. St. Louis: C.V. Mosby Co., 1978.

Miller, Benjamin F., and Claire B. Keane. ENCYCLOPEDIA AND DICTIONARY OF MEDICINE AND NURSING. Philadelphia: W.B. Saunders Co., 1972.

Moore, Mary L. REALITIES IN CHILDBEARING. Philadelphia: W.B. Saunders Co., 1978.

Oaks, Wilbur W., ed. CRITICAL CARE MEDICINE. (The Twenty Eighth Hahnemann Symposium) New York: Grune & Stratton, 1974.

Oxorn, H., and W.R. Foote. HUMAN LABOR AND BIRTH, 3rd ed. New York: Appleton-Century-Crofts, 1975.

Pritchard, J.A., and P.C. MacDonald. WILLIAMS OBSTETRICS, 15th ed. New York: Appleton-Century-Crofts, 1976.

Roberts, Florence B. PERINATAL NURSING: CARE OF NEWBORNS AND THEIR FAMILIES. New York: McGraw-Hill Book Co., 1977.

Schroeder, John S., and Elaine K. Daily. TECHNIQUES IN BEDSIDE HEMODYNAMIC MONITORING. St. Louis: C.V. Mosby Co., 1976.

Shapiro, Barry A., et al. CLINICAL APPLICATION OF BLOOD GASES, 2nd ed. Chicago: Year Book Medical Publishers, Inc., 1977.

Shires, George T., ed. CARE OF THE TRAUMA PATIENT, 2nd ed. New York: McGraw-Hill Book Co., 1979.

Spivak, Jerry L., and H. Verdain Barnes. MANUAL OF CLINICAL PROBLEMS IN INTERNAL MEDICINE. Boston: Little, Brown & Co., 1978.

Taber, B. MANUAL OF GYNECOLOGIC AND OBSTETRIC EMERGENCIES. Philadelphia: W.B. Saunders Co., 1979.

Tucker, S.M., and S. Bryant. FETAL MONITORING AND FETAL ASSESSMENT IN HIGH RISK PREGNANCY. St. Louis: C.V. Mosby Co., 1978.

Whaley, L., and D. Wong. NURSING CARE OF INFANTS AND CHILDREN. St. Louis: C.V. Mosby Co., 1979.

Wilkins, Earl W., Jr., ed. MGH TEXTBOOK OF EMERGENCY MEDICINE: EMERGENCY CARE AS PRACTICED AT THE MASSACHUSETTS GENERAL HOSPITAL. Baltimore: Williams & Wilkins Co., 1978.

Ziegel, E., and C. Van Blarcom. OBSTETRIC NURSING, 7th ed. New York: Macmillan Publishing Co., 1978.

Periodicals

Finnegan, L., and B. MacNew. *Care of the addicted infant,* AMERICAN JOURNAL OF NURSING. 74:685-93, April 1974.

Fulton, R.L. "Trauma," The University of Louisville School of Medicine Symposium. *Penetrating wounds of the heart,* HEART & LUNG. 7:262-268, March/April 1978.

Jennings, B. *Emergency delivery: How to attend to one safely,* AMERICAN JOURNAL OF MATERNAL CHILD NURSING. 4:148-153, May/June 1979.

Kantor, G.K. *Addicted mother, addicted baby: A challenge to health care providers,* Part 2, THE AMERICAN JOURNAL OF MATERNAL CHILD NURSING. 3:281-285, September/October 1978.

Nalepka, C.D. *The oxygen hood for newborns in respiratory distress,* AMERICAN JOURNAL OF NURSING. 75:2185-2187, December 1975.

Oakes, G.K., R.A. Chez, and I.C. Morelli. *Diet in pregnancy: Meddling with the normal or preventing toxemia?* AMERICAN JOURNAL OF NURSING. 75:1134-1136, July 1975.

Richardson, J.D. "Trauma," The University of Louisville School of Medicine Symposium. *Management of noncardiac thoracic trauma,* HEART & LUNG. 7:286-292, March/April, 1978.

Skillman, T.G. "Endocrine and metabolic emergencies," The Ohio State University. *Diabetic ketoacidosis,* Part 2, HEART & LUNG. 7:594-602, July/August 1978.

Index